Teaching Resources for End-of-Life and Palliative Care Courses

Also Available from Lyceum Books, Inc.

Advisory Editor: Thomas M. Meenaghan, *New York University*

ETHICS IN END-OF-LIFE DECISIONS FOR SOCIAL WORK PRACTICE,
by Ellen Csikai and Elizabeth Chaiten

A PRACTICAL GUIDE TO SOCIAL SERVICE EVALUATION,
by Carl F. Brun

ENDINGS IN CLINICAL PRACTICE: EFFECTIVE CLOSURE IN DIVERSE SETTINGS, 2E,
by Joseph Walsh, foreword by Thomas M. Meenaghan

SECONDARY TRAUMATIC STRESS AND THE CHILD WELFARE PROFESSIONAL,
by Josephine G. Pryce, Kimberly K. Shackelford, and David H. Pryce

STRAIGHT TALK ABOUT PROFESSIONAL ETHICS,
by Kim Strom-Gottfried

WHAT IS PROFESSIONAL SOCIAL WORK?,
by Malcolm Payne

USING STATISTICAL METHODS IN SOCIAL WORK PRACTICE WITH SPSS,
by Soleman H. Abu-Bader

EVIDENCE-BASED PRACTICES FOR SOCIAL WORKERS,
by Thomas O'Hare

SHORT-TERM EXISTENTIAL INTERVENTION IN CLINICAL PRACTICE,
by Jim Lantz and Joseph Walsh

CLINICAL ASSESSMENT FOR SOCIAL WORKERS: QUALITATIVE AND QUANTITATIVE METHODS, 2E,
edited by Catheleen Jordan and Cynthia Franklin

TEAMWORK IN MULTIPROFESSIONAL CARE,
by Malcolm Payne, foreword by Thomas M. Meenaghan

ADVOCACY PRACTICE FOR SOCIAL JUSTICE,
by Richard Hoefer

Teaching Resources for End-of-Life and Palliative Care Courses

Edited by

Ellen L. Csikai
University of Alabama

Barbara Jones
University of Texas–Austin

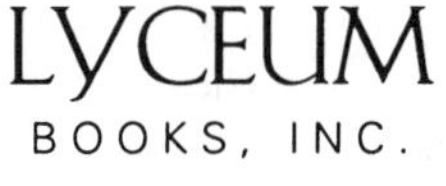

Chicago, Illinois

Published by
LYCEUM BOOKS, INC.
5758 S. Blackstone Ave.
Chicago, Illinois 60637
773+643-1903 (Fax)
773+643-1902 (Phone)
lyceum@lyceumbooks.com
http://www.lyceumbooks.com

10 9 8 7 6 5 4 3 2 1
ISBN 978-1-933478-10-4

Library of Congress Cataloging-in-Publication Data

Teaching resources for end-of-life and palliative care courses / [edited by] Ellen L. Csikai, Barbara Jones.
p. cm.
Includes bibliographical references.
ISBN-13: 978-1-933478-09-8 (electronic format)
ISBN-13: 978-1-933478-10-4 (alk. paper)
1. Medical social work—Study and teaching. 2. Palliative treatment—Study and teaching. 3. Social education—Curricula. I. Csikai, Ellen L. II. Jones, Barbara.
HV687.T43 2007
362.17'5071—dc22

2007005713

Contents

Preface

End-of-life care issues are encountered by social workers in all areas of practice. In health-care settings these can be seen in hospitals and in hospices, nursing homes, and outpatient clinics. Helping individuals and families cope with a newly diagnosed life-limiting illness, a chronic debilitating illness, or the terminal stages of illness, social workers assist people when they are most vulnerable. In other settings, for example, in child protective services, social workers may encounter a grandparent caring for a dependent child whose mother died from complications of AIDS. In schools, social workers may attend to the mental health of classmates of a student who was killed in a car crash or has committed suicide.

The limited current research and literature in end-of-life care in social work has indicated that health-care social workers are not as prepared as they need to be or would like to be in working with end-of-life care issues (Christ & Sormanti, 1999; Csikai & Bass, 2000; Kovacs & Bronstein, 1999). Also, hospice social workers have identified cross-disciplinary training and collaboration as important in providing a holistic approach in end-of-life care (Kovacs & Bronstein, 1999). Health-care social workers attending a seminar providing training in end-of-life care issues agreed that end-of-life concerns are growing in number and intensity, and they believed that there was a need for ongoing discussion, education, and guidance as to how to best handle these situations (Csikai & Bass, 2000).

The curricula required by the Council on Social Work Education in BSW and MSW programs prepare social workers to assist in enhancing the well-being of individuals and families in a variety of settings through comprehensive assessment and multi-modal treatment. However, specific information related to end-of-life care presented in most BSW and MSW training programs is limited. Resources for social work faculty for teaching content in end-of-life care have been limited as well. In a comprehensive review of fifty social work textbooks, Kramer, Hovland-Scafe, and Pacourek (2003) reported that of 19,377 pages of text, only 651 pages (3.35%) were related to end-of-life care. The development and institutionalization of social work education for work with the dying is necessary for the profession in order for social workers to competently fulfill the recently formulated (2004) *NASW Standards for Social Work Practice in Palliative and End-of-Life Care* and work toward improving care at the end of life.

We believe that offering a comprehensive resource to social work educators at all levels will begin to fill the gap in knowledge about end-of-life care and how best to incorporate this content into social work programs.

REFERENCES

Christ, G. H., & Sormanti, M. (1999). Advancing social work practice in end-of-life care. *Social Work in Health Care, 30*(2), 81–99.

Csikai, E. L., & Bass, K. (2000). Health care social workers' views of ethical issues, practice, and policy in end-of-life care. *Social Work in Health Care, 32*(2), 1–22.

Kovacs, P., & Bronstein, L. (1999). Preparation for oncology settings: What hospice social workers say they need. *Social Work in Health Care, 24*(1), 57–64.

Kramer, B. J., Hovland-Scafe, C., & Pacourek, L. (2003). Analysis of end-of-life content in social work textbooks. *Journal of Social Work Education, 39*(2), 299–320.

National Association of Social Workers. (2004). *NASW standards for social work practice in palliative and end-of-life care.* Retrieved from http://www.naswdc.org/practice/bereavement/standards/default.asp

ACKNOWLEDGMENTS

The editors wish to thank all those who submitted materials for this compendium. We believe all contributions served to make this a quality resource. We would also like to thank Laurel Hitchcock and Hae Jung Shin, graduate research assistants and PhD students in the School of Social Work at the University of Alabama, for their assistance in coordinating submissions and the initial formatting and editing of the manuscript.

Introduction

This compendium is intended to be a resource for new faculty with an interest in end-of-life care, and for seasoned faculty who wish to update their current courses or take on a new area of teaching. Also, it will provide concrete guidance for adjunct or part-time faculty who are practitioners in end-of-life care settings that will add academic rigor to the rich experience they bring to the classroom

In this book, we have compiled resources that we believe provide a comprehensive view of content that is currently being taught in end-of-life care at the undergraduate and masters levels as well as in continuing education and post-masters training. It turned out that it was not an easy feat to put this book of resources together because teaching about end-of-life care has evolved in recent years to encompass more than traditional death-and-dying or grief-and-bereavement courses. It didn't take too many submissions to show us the diversity of social work education in end-of-life care that is taking place.

The first section contains a listing of books serving as primary textbooks and a listing of recommended books for the courses. The recommended book list was compiled from all syllabi that were submitted (not only from the syllabi that we included in this book). Books that are listed on both the primary textbook list and the recommended book list are marked by an asterisk.

The next section consists of assessment tools that can be used by practitioners with clients. They can be used in the classroom as self-reflective exercises or for students to practice through role-playing. The first, a special submission from Garthwait, introduces us to a life review tool. It is an event life review called "A Century in Review," which she developed with the support grant funding from the John A. Hartford Foundation. We thank her for sharing this and allowing it to be published in this book. At the end of life and during the bereavement process, spirituality and meaning in life often become very important. Murdock provides us with tools that can be shared with practitioners and students to facilitate a thorough assessment of spirituality issues in older populations.

The next two sections contain compilations of self-reflective exercises and class assignments. In particular we thought it was important to stress the value of self-reflective exercises for use in social work courses, as students must examine their own personal beliefs and values so that their practice with individuals who are dying or bereaved may reach its fullest potential. Many of the syllabi included in this book provide additional exercises and assignments that do not appear in these two sections; please also see these syllabi for examples of other self-reflective exercises and course assignments.

The next four sections contain exemplary syllabi and are divided into four categories: BSW courses, MSW courses on end-of-life care—comprehensive/ life-span content; MSW courses on loss, grief, and bereavement; and MSW specialty courses

We were pleased to have a number of submissions for BSW courses that provide a solid foundation for practice at the bachelors level. End-of-life care and grief-and-loss issues are present in every practice setting, and thus every social worker needs a minimum level of knowledge and skill in this area. The syllabi from Manfred-Gilham, Roff, and Roth are examples of end-of-life care from a generalist perspective. In addition, the five course modules developed by Brandsen and Carlsen for educating generalist practitioners can stand alone as distinct units or may be used to incorporate grief and end-of-life content into more general BSW courses.

Since the MSW syllabi submitted represented a broad range of topics, we tried to organize them into distinct categories. The first MSW syllabus section contains exemplary syllabi that contain comprehensive content in end-of-life care. This means that content on aspects of dying; definitions; cultural, religious, and spiritual perspectives; legal and ethical issues; and grief and bereavement issues are presented. They provide an overall view of content needed for social work practice with end-of-life issues. Contributors here are Csikai, Linder, Lindhorst and Letinich, Sanders, and Schroepfer. Of particular interest may be the Linder syllabus, which describes an interdisciplinary course aimed at students in both social work and divinity studies.

The second section of MSW syllabi contains syllabi that focus more specifically on loss, grief, and bereavement. Even within this section a range of topics across the life span are covered in the courses contributed by Becvar, De St. Aubin, Green, Kramer, Walsh, and Walsh-Burke. Of particular interest may be the grief-and-loss course taught by Walsh-Burke totally online.

The third section of MSW syllabi covers a range of specialized topics. Some of these courses are focused on specialized areas within end-of-life care, such as Jones's Pediatric Palliative and End-of-Life Care, an empirically based curriculum based on a research conducted with support from Project on Death in America, and Miller's End-of-Life Decision Making. Others are specialized courses that, due to the nature of the substantive area, necessitate course content specific to end-of-life care, such as Bern-Klug's Introduction to Nursing Homes and Taylor-Brown's AIDS and Social Work Practice: Policy and Practice Issues. These syllabi all reveal a unique approach to the inclusion of end-of-life care content in graduate social work education.

The next section contains information on four specialty programs. The end-of-life care field of practice that is offered at the University of Iowa is also a resource for MSW programs. The program was developed by Murty, with the support of a Project on Death in America Social Work Leadership Development Award. What is unique about this field of practice is the focus on end-of-life care in rural communities. The continuing education workshop developed by Liley gives a unique approach to providing end-of-life care and grief-and-loss content to practitioners. It utilizes an intensive-weekend teaching format and includes content of a wide range of end-of-life topic areas. Finally, the end-of-life care certificate program offered by Baystate Medical Center in Northampton, Massachusetts (developed through Smith College School for Social Work by Berzoff), and the New York University end-of-life certificate program (developed by Dane, professor emerita) are post-master's programs developed with funding support from the Project on Death in America Social Work Leadership Development Award. They provide advanced clinical content for practitioners who are or wish to specialize in end-of-life care practice.

The final section contains other resources that may be useful to both educators and practitioners. An Internet resource developed by Bullock (also with Project on Death in America Social Work Leadership Development Award support) is described. The site is maintained through the School of Social Work at the University of Connecticut and provides an end-of-life information clearinghouse. The second entry is a current list of end-of-life resources offered by the National Association of Social Workers.

We think that you will agree that this resource book is truly that! We hope that you will find many items that are useful as you design courses in end-of-life care, palliative care, and grief and bereavement.

Part One

Textbooks

1

Primary Textbooks

Albom, M. (1997). *Tuesdays with Morrie.* New York: Bantam Doubleday Dell.*

This book is a chronicle of the time that was spent together by a young man (Mitch) and his mentor/professor from years ago (Morrie). The relationship between the two men was rekindled after many years had passed. Mitch graduated from college and is now involved in his own life. Time goes by. As he flips through TV channels, he sees Morrie on an edition of *Nightline* with Ted Koppel. Morrie is on the program to talk about living and dying with ALS. Mitch makes the decision to visit his old mentor/professor, and they decide to chronicle their visits as a lesson on life, dying, and death. The book deals with how individuals face impending death, the importance of human relationships, and the idea of learning how to live while one is dying. Students have said that this is not a book that they would have read if it had not been assigned. They are generally very happy that they have read this book; in fact, many tell me that it has changed the way they approach conversations about dying and death with other people. Some have said that this book has changed their lives.

Becvar, D. S. (2001). *In the presence of grief: Helping family members successfully resolve death, dying and bereavement issues.* New York: Guilford Press.

This book addresses various grief-related issues, including understanding death, dying, and bereavement; when death comes unannounced; when death is anticipated; the question of euthanasia; when a child dies; when a sibling dies; when a parent dies; when a spouse dies; and when an extended family member or friend dies. Also considered is grief in the context of therapy, including creating funerals and other healing rituals, searching for meaning, and reclaiming joy. Each chapter is introduced with a story derived from the personal experience of one of the contributors and ends with a clinical vignette derived from the professional experience of the author.

Behrman, G. (2004). *The invisible people: How the U.S. has slept through the global AIDS pandemic, the greatest humanitarian catastrophe of our time.* New York: Free Press.

This book reports on the global AIDS crisis and examines the policies of power and privilege underlying the lack of an effective U.S. response to the AIDS pandemic. Behrman describes what he calls "one of the deadliest policy failures in the history of the U.S. government" and issues a call to action for those who advocate for the disenfranchised people of the world.

Berzoff, J., & Silverman, P. (2004). *Living with dying: A handbook for end-of-life healthcare practitioners.* New York: Columbia University Press.*

Living with Dying begins with the narratives of five health-care professionals who, when faced with overwhelming personal losses, altered their clinical practices and philosophies. The book discusses ways to ensure a respectful death for individuals; speaks to families, groups, and communities; and is organized around clinical practice with individuals, families, and groups. The book addresses practice with people who have illnesses such as AIDS, bone marrow disease, and cancer and pays special attention to patients who have been stigmatized due to culture, ability, sexual orientation, age, race, or homelessness. The book includes content on trauma and developmental issues for children, adults, and older individuals who are dying, and it addresses legal, ethical, spiritual, cultural, and social class issues as core factors in the assessment of and work with the dying. It explores interdisciplinary teamwork, supervision, and the organizational and financial context in which dying occurs. Current research in end-of-life care; ways to provide leadership in the field; and a call for compassion, insight, and respect for the dying complete this book.

This is a comprehensive resource on end-of-life care that is aimed particularly at social workers in this field of practice. Many of the chapters are written by social workers in both academia and the practice world. The chapters are accessible and easy to read. Many chapters utilize concrete case examples to aid teaching and understanding of the material. It is an excellent book to use in MSW courses designed to cover many end-of-life topics across the life span.

Byock, I. (1997). *Dying well: Peace and possibilities at the end of life.* New York: Riverhead Books.

This book was chosen for a course because it has the power of stories. The many narratives in the book touch on a wide range of topics, including suffering, pain, letting go, loss, acceptance, and opportunity. Told from the viewpoint of a physician, this material allows students to explore difficult topics in an informal way. The accounts of patient and family experiences in the book can be tied to the didactic material offered in the classroom.

Callanan, M., & Kelley, P. (1997). *Final gifts: Understanding the special awareness, needs, and communications of the dying*. New York: Bantam Books.

Final Gifts provides an insider's view of the dying process from the perspective of two hospice nurses. Callanan and Kelley document the spiritual, psychological, emotional, cognitive, and physical journey that multiple patients travel as they enter the final days of their lives. These case studies provide the reader with detailed information about the dying process and how many hospice patients provide their family members with clues to their dying experience. This book is a favorite in my death-and-dying class because it allows the students to slowly unwrap some of the mystery of the dying process and demonstrates the peace that many people find in their final days.

Corr, C. A., Nabe, C. M., & Corr, D. M. (2003). *Death and dying: Life and living*. Belmont, CA: Wadsworth/Thomson Learning.

This book helps to provide an understanding of dying, death, and bereavement that will assist individuals in better coping with their own death and the deaths of others. It is a book that offers an understanding of what it means to have experienced the dying and death of a loved one or of someone who is entrusted to one's professional care. What is particularly unique about this text is its usefulness for a classroom setting. At the end of each chapter, questions are presented for discussion and in-class assignments. The text also comes with an instructor's manual and test bank. Grief and bereavement are discussed in this book as psychological processes that must be handled with sensitivity. All topics related to dying and death, life and living, are presented with appropriate references and an updated bibliography.

Csikai, E. L., & Chaitin, E. (2005). *Ethics in end-of-life decisions in social work practice*. Chicago: Lyceum Books.

Ethics in End-of-Life Decisions in Social Work Practice provides a comprehensive and practical approach to understanding end-of-life decisions. The authors connect long-standing philosophical theories to contemporary concerns in the field of bioethics. Topics covered are bioethical principles and key issues related to the end of life and ethical decisions in health care, including clinical decision-making processes and privacy and confidentiality. Also covered is how to assess capacity for decision making and design treatment and intervention plans in coordination with health-care teams. The authors include case studies to show the complex end-of-life decisions faced by patients, families, and health-care workers. Approaches are offered for resolving debates about informed consent, privacy and confidentiality, and the refusal or denial of medical treatment. This book provides the practical knowledge that social workers need for effective practice with clients facing end-of-life decisions. It also provides the knowledge social workers need to fully participate in interdisciplinary health-care team discussions of these important issues. Students will find the information easy to read and to apply to their future practice.

DeSpelder, L., & Strickland, A. (Eds.). (2005). *The last dance: Encountering death and dying* (7th ed.). Boston: McGraw-Hill.

This is a new edition of a well-known introductory text that is often used in the field. The book provides an interdisciplinary and cross-cultural examination of issues related to death, dying, and bereavement. Included are surveys of attitudes toward death, historical perspectives, discussions of health-care systems, cultural traditions regarding funerals and bereavement, medical ethics, and the law, as well as death in the lives of children.

Fadiman, A. (1998). *The spirit catches you and you fall down*. New York: Farrar, Straus and Giroux.

This book provides a look at issues of life, health care, and death as they are experienced by the Hmong people living in America. The author recounts the story of Lia Lee, the daughter of Hmong immigrants who believe her seizures were caused by the slamming of a door that made her soul flee her body. The resulting cultural clash between the American health-care system and Lia's Hmong family is an excellent example of the often-neglected and difficult-to-resolve issues of cultural self-determination versus the medical model.

Hooyman, N. R., & Kramer, B. J. (2005). *Living through loss: Interventions across the lifespan*. New York: Columbia University Press.

Living through Loss: Interventions across the Lifespan highlights the wide range and types of losses encountered across the life span and profiles developmentally congruent and evidence-based interventions. In this way it is a very useful resource for a grief class because it helps social work students understand the causes and conditions that give rise to grief and what they might do in practice to respond appropriately. The text explores the nature and centrality of the experience of loss encountered in practice very broadly and discusses death- and nondeath-related losses (e.g., giving birth to a child with disabilities; living with chronic illness; going through a divorce; being assaulted, abused, or otherwise traumatized). Initial chapters provide a comprehensive review of the historical and contemporary theoretical perspectives on grief and the grief process and put forth a resiliency model for understanding personal, family, social, and cultural capacities that affect grief and other outcomes of loss at each developmental life phase. This is followed by chapters examining loss at five phases of the life span (childhood, adolescence, young adulthood, midlife, and later life) and corresponding chapters on developmentally appropriate interventions to address these losses at the individual, family, group, and community levels. Attention is given to the role of age, race, culture, sexual orientation, gender, and spirituality in a person's response to loss. Finally, the gifts and challenges experienced by professionals who bear witness to the suffering of their clients are reviewed, along with suggestions for self-awareness and self-care.

Institute of Medicine. (2003). *When children die: Improving palliative and end-of-life care for children and their families.* Washington, DC: National Academies Press.

This book documents the experiences of children with life-threatening illnesses and their families in the U.S. health-care system. Strategies for improving the care of these children are presented, including policy, education, and practice recommendations. Future research needs are also discussed. The Institute for Medicine initiated the study and collected information from professionals as well as from parents and professional groups.

Irish, D. P., Lundquist, K. F., & Nelson, V. J. (Eds.). (1993). *Ethnic variations in dying, death and grief: Diversity in universality.* Washington, DC: Taylor and Francis.*

This book is a compilation of in-depth articles intended to help those working in occupations related to death and dying work more effectively with clients from diverse social and ethnic groups. It provides illustrative examples of ethnic patterns and materials about death and dying and multicultural issues. Each of the chapters was written by specialists from various backgrounds who share the cultural traditions they describe and examines how each culture looks at death and dying. The book acknowledges that groups are not homogeneous within themselves, and individual variation must always be taken into account. It also contains a self-assessment tool for cultural readiness and awareness.

Kastenbaum, R. J. (2004). *Death, society, and human experience* (8th ed.). Needham Heights, MA: Allyn and Bacon.

Death, Society, and Human Experience provides a thorough overview of death-related topics and is appropriate for undergraduate survey courses in death, dying, and bereavement. Death is approached from both macro (the death system, policy choices) and micro (personal experiences with death, the grieving process) perspectives. Chapters focus on children and death, end-of-life care, suicide, and funeral processes. Each chapter includes exercises and case examples. The book coordinates well with the series *Death: A Personal Understanding,* produced by the Annenberg/CPB project. The films in this series are excellent for class discussions.

Kissane, D. W., & Bloch, S. (2003). *Family focused grief therapy.* Philadelphia: Open University Press.

This book focuses on the family as the unit of care during the dying process. The authors present a model of family care that includes techniques for supporting both the patient and family members during the palliative care experience, death, and bereavement. A step-by-step approach to assessment and intervention is outlined.

Leming, M. R., & Dickinson, G. E. (2002). *Understanding dying, death, and bereavement* (5th ed.). Fort Worth, TX: Harcourt College.

This book takes a social-psychological theory and research approach to the subjects of dying, death, and bereavement. The fifth edition places greater emphasis on individual coping with death and dying, particularly through the use of personal narratives integrated throughout the text. Social-psychological concepts are applied to specific narrative examples. Cross-cultural perspectives are included, with a special emphasis on how they influence rituals of death and dying.

Mappes, T. A., & DeGrazia, D. (2001). *Biomedical ethics* (5th ed.). Boston: McGraw-Hill.

This anthology of case studies and readings connects ethical issues in medicine to the practice of health care today. Conflicts of interest, advance directives, physician-assisted suicide, and the allocation of health care are some of the topics examined.

Neimeyer, R. (2002). *Meaning and reconstruction and the experience of loss* (2nd ed.). Washington, DC: American Psychological Association.*

The main concept in *Meaning Reconstruction and the Experience of Loss* is that loss is not loss is not loss. This collection of seventeen texts by psychotherapists, psychologists, and religious scholars makes clear that death does not in itself constitute loss or trigger debilitating grief, but that it challenges survivors to engage in a complex process of constructing meaning. These constructions may include a sense of hopelessness, fear, and remorse. However, the author's uplifting message is that loss may be reconstructed in myriad ways that go beyond the negative. Many of these chapters emphasize the meaning-making process as inherently a social one. Whether relying on social traditions or ongoing relationships, making meaning is not a private but a cultural activity. The importance of family and communal relations in reconstructing loss is examined.

Pequegnat, W., & Szapocznik, J. (Eds.). (2000). *Working with families in the era of HIV/AIDS*. Thousand Oaks, CA: Sage.

Working with families in the era of HIV/AIDS encourages families to become involved in preventing the spread of HIV. The book provides examples of strategies for mobilizing family resources in the prevention of HIV and AIDS, as well as family-oriented adaptation strategies for living with the disease. Promising prevention strategies identified by the NIMH Consortium on Families and HIV/AIDS are presented. The approaches, which have been specifically developed for use among African American families, are currently being tested in controlled trials across the country.

Quill, T. (2001). *Caring for patients at the end of life: Facing an uncertain future together*. New York: Oxford University Press.

Quill's book includes chapters covering several important issues: nonabandonment, delivering bad news, palliative care for patients with severe dementia, and double effect. The book has helpful tables that assist with the formulation of assessment questions around difficult topics. There is also valuable information on how to negotiate differences and conflict around end-of-life decisions. This book also offers guidance on how to explore requests for assistance with death.

Rantz, M. J., & Flesner, M. K. (2004). *Person centered care: A model for nursing homes*. Washington, DC: American Nurses Association

This soft-cover booklet introduces the reader to some of the problems facing nursing homes and how one nursing home, Crestview Home in Bethany, Missouri, has overcome many of these problems. The booklet describes the professional context of person-centered care, the benefits of implementing "person care" for residents and staff, and how different departments are affected. There is a helpful appendix with copies of the actual forms developed and used at Crestview Home, including the Wants and Desires form, the Life History Form, the Do-You-Like-It-Here checklist, and the room checklist. The booklet is easy to read and inspires nursing homes and broader society to reconsider underlying assumptions about the provision of care. It suggests placing more emphasis on enhancing resident quality of life, as defined by each resident.

Rantz, M., Popejoy, L., & Zwygart-Stauffacher, M. (2001). *The new nursing homes: A 20-minute way to find great long-term care.* Minneapolis, MN: Fairview Press.

This 170-page soft-cover book provides a wealth of information about how to gauge the care and quality of life at a nursing home. The book contains many checklists and much advice that families can use as they walk through a nursing home and interview staff and family members of residents. Social work students have shared that they find the book useful as a starting place to talk with families about how to visit a nursing home with open eyes.

Sprang, G., & McNeil, J. (1995). *The many faces of bereavement: The nature and treatment of natural, traumatic, and stigmatized grief.* New York: Brunner/Mazel.

This book presents a theoretical overview of traditional models of grief response. Examples include the grief response to spousal death (with a focus on the elderly), parental grief following the loss of a child, traumatic grief, grief following community disaster, and grief following stigmatized death such as suicide or HIV/AIDS.

Viorst, J. (1986). *Necessary losses.* New York: Simon and Schuster.

Redbook columnist Judith Viorst combines personal experience, psychoanalytic theory, and knowledge of the literature to make the case that growing and aging involve a succession of conscious and unconscious losses. The loss of the mother-child connection, youth, and our loved ones through separation and death are all experiences that Viorst identifies as necessary for gaining greater wisdom about life.

Walsh, F. (2006). *Strengthening family resilience* (2nd ed.). New York: Guilford Press.

This revised and updated edition expands Walsh's family resilience framework for working with families experiencing adversity. The author draws on clinical experience and research to describe key processes for helping families develop resiliency to a range of challenges, including trauma, loss, and serious illness.

Walsh, F., & McGoldrick, M. (2006). *Living beyond loss: Death in the family* (2nd ed.). New York: W. W. Norton.

This book examines the impact of death on the family system. Therapeutic guidelines are presented for helping families work through the mourning process. This new edition includes discussions of spirituality, traumatic death, and stigmatized losses and how they affect the family system. A new section offers personal reflections by prominent family therapists regarding loss and bereavement.

Walsh-Burke, K. (2006). *Grief and loss: Theories and skills for helping professionals.* Needham Heights, MA: Allyn and Bacon.

The author provides case studies to illustrate theories and skills for strengthening the response of helping professionals to patients and clients experiencing grief and loss. Key concepts relevant to everyday practice are discussed, and student exercises suitable for in-class activities or independent assignments are included.

Worden, J. W. (2002). *Grief counseling and grief therapy: A handbook for the mental health practitioner* (3rd ed.). New York: Springer.*

This book draws on research, clinical practice, and the literature to discuss death and bereavement. The four tasks of mourning are outlined, as are the seven mediators of mourning.

Working Committee on HIV, Children and Families. (1996). *Families in crisis: Report of the Working Committee on HIV, Children and Families.* New York: Federation of Protestant Social Workers.

In 1995, the New York State Legislature requested that the AIDS Institute of the New York State Department of Health, in conjunction with other relevant agencies and service providers, produce a report on children orphaned by HIV/AIDS and a plan for comprehensive permanency planning in New York State. Substantial increases in the rates of HIV infection among women in New York and a consequent near doubling of the estimated number of children and adolescents who will be orphaned by maternal HIV/AIDS death by the beginning of the century have created an increased need for services. The Working Committee on HIV, Children and Families was convened to develop this report and make recommendations.

Wyatt-Morley, C. (1997). *AIDS memoir: Journal of an HIV-positive mother.* West Hartford, CT: Kumarian Press.

The author uses journal entries to recount her journey of living with AIDS in middle-class America as a woman of color. Divorce, job discrimination, isolation, declining physical health, and family refusal to deal with the illness are all discussed as Wyatt-Worley struggles to document for her children the reality of fighting both the disease and the system.

2

Recommended Books

Albom, M. (1997). *Tuesdays with Morrie*. New York: Bantam Doubleday Dell.*

Berzoff, J., & Silverman, P. (2004). *Living with dying: A handbook for end-of-life healthcare practitioners*. New York: Columbia University Press.*

Callahan, B. N. (1999). *Grief counseling: A manual for social workers*. Denver, CO: Love Publishing.

Crosson-Tower, C. (2003). *From the eye of the storm: The experiences of a child welfare worker*. Needham Heights, MA: Allyn and Bacon.

Farmer, P., Connors, M., & Simmons, J. (2005). *Women, poverty, and AIDS*. Boston: Common Courage Press.

Fry, V. (1995). *Part of me died too: Stories of creative survival among bereaved children and teenagers*. New York: Dutton Children's Books.

Gunther, J. (1998). *Death be not proud*. New York: Harper Perennial Classics.

Irish, D. P., Lundquist, K. F., & Nelson, V. J. (Eds.). (1993). *Ethnic variations in dying, death and grief: Diversity in universality*. Washington, DC: Taylor and Francis.*

Krementz, J. (1988). *How it feels when a parent dies*. New York: Knopf.

Lerner, G. (1978). *A death of one's own*. New York: Harper and Row.

Mannino, J. D. (1997). *Grieving days, healing days*. Needham Heights, MA: Allyn and Bacon.

McGoldrick, M. (1991). *Living beyond loss*. London: W. W. Norton.

Neimeyer, R. (2002). *Meaning and reconstruction and the experience of loss* (2nd ed.). Washington, DC: American Psychological Association.*

Parry, J. K., & Ryan, A. S. (Eds.). (1995). *A cross-cultural look at death, dying and religion*. Chicago: Nelson-Hall.

Rando, T. A. (1984). *Grief, dying and death*. Champaign, IL: Research Press.

Rando, T. A. (Ed.). (1986). *Parental loss of a child*. Champaign, IL: Research Press.

Rando, T. A. (1998). *Treatment of complicated mourning*. Champaign, IL: Research Press.*

Rolland, J. R. (1994). *Families, illness, and disability: An integrative treatment model*. New York: Basic Books.

Roth, P. (1993). *Patrimony.* New York: Random House.

Tolstoy, L. (1960). *The death of Ivan Ilych.* New York: New American Library.

Walsh, F. (Ed.). (1999). *Spiritual resources in family therapy.* New York: Guilford Press.

Walsh, F. (Ed.). (2003). *Normal family processes: Growing diversity and complexity* (3rd ed.). New York: Guilford Press.

Worden, J. W. (1996). *Children and grief.* New York: Guilford Press.

Worden, J. W. (2002). *Grief counseling and grief therapy: A handbook for the mental health practitioner* (3rd ed.). New York: Springer.*

Part Two

Assessment Tools

3

A Century in Review

A Decade-by-Decade Social and Historical Timeline

Cynthia Garthwait

INTRODUCTION

Social workers pride themselves on their natural and professionally acquired skills in communication. We claim to be able to relate to a wide variety of people, most of them quite different from ourselves. While this is true, it is also important to recognize the challenges of getting beyond the constraints of the context of one's own sociohistorical place in time. If we do not understand how the filters and lenses through which we see the world limit our ability to understand those with whom we work, we may never truly understand another's life fully, if we ever can. What then can we do to equip ourselves to see older adults as they see themselves and to understand the uniqueness of their lives? What tools might we add to our repertoire of skills in addition to our desire to relate to older people? A mere study of history itself will not allow us a meaningful glimpse into our clients' lives. Instead, perhaps what is needed is a way to bring to life the stories set in time.

USING THE TOOLS

This collection of tools is designed to assist in conducting meaningful social assessments of elders by providing templates that can guide interviews with older adults. When interviewing your elder, you can use these templates (1) to organize and prepare for the time you spend together, (2) to encourage reflection by your elder on his or her life as set in a sociohistorical context, and (3) to examine the social justice issues experienced firsthand by your elder over his or her life span. One of the most positive potential outcomes of life review for elders is the weaving together of the strands of their lives, building upon the private life review in which they may already be engaged individually. Your skills and contribution toward helping them through a life review set in time may result in a number of positive outcomes for elders:

- You may help them view their lives in a more favorable light than they were able to do alone.
- You may help them resolve issues with which they have struggled for a long time, and with which they still struggle.
- You may help them make more meaning of their lives.

This is a shared journey on which you are invited to embark, and for which I hope you are grateful to be included. Both you and your elder should gain a new perspective on life, on social justice, and on the richness of life that can be had when one generation touches another.

Life Review/Reminiscence Questions to Stimulate Discussion of Social Justice between Elder and Student

Did your family feel protected by the laws in effect while you were a child?

How were girls and boys raised differently when you were a child?

What advantages do your grandchildren have that you did not?

How have their lives been different as a result?

Were you ever limited in your lifetime due to income, gender, or ethnicity?

What major historical events affected your life the most?

Did you participate in politics in order to change unjust laws?

If you could talk to anyone in history, who would it be?

If you could live in any era, which would it be?

What do today's young people take for granted that you did not have?

What social programs that exist now would have improved your earlier life had they been in existence when you were younger (unemployment insurance, health-care coverage, civil rights, social security, family planning)?

How did families deal with issues like poverty?

When do you first remember the government taking responsibility for such issues as unemployment, poverty, health care, workers' rights, family planning, and race relations?

What experiences with discrimination shaped your life in both negative and positive ways?

What major social injustices did you see addressed during your lifetime?

Is social justice viewed the same way today as it was viewed when you were younger?

Critical Thinking Questions and Assignments for Student Analysis and Reflection on Social Justice

How might events and social policies during the years when your client was a child have affected his or her development?

How can Erik Erikson's model of psychosocial development be combined with an understanding of historical/cultural events and social policy to help you better understand your client?

What impact did the lack of programs and services we take for granted today (i.e., health insurance, retirement pensions, birth control, civil rights protection, unemployment insurance) have on your client's life?

Compare benefits and protections available to a woman in 1920 with those available to a woman in 2007. How have they changed? How might her life have been different if those benefits had been available to her and her family earlier in life?

How did the shift from family responsibility for social welfare to governmental responsibility for social safety nets affect family life in the United States?

Examine the social policies and programs available to your client during adolescence and young adulthood. Compare them with social policies and programs available to you during your adolescence and young adulthood. How are your life experiences different as a result?

How does the experience of privilege (having benefits that others do not have) affect your ability to understand your clients who did not have these benefits during their lifetime?

How can understanding the sociohistorical context of your clients' lives enhance your ability to provide services to them?

Study a social issue such as health care, civil rights, gender issues, mental health, or poverty through the twentieth century. Learn how historical events, cultural shifts, societal attitudes, and social policies changed the ways in which individuals and families experienced those social issues over time.

1900–1909

Social and Historical Timeline		*Client Timeline*
1900	Yellow Fever Commission formed	
1900	Harry Houdini popular in Europe	
1901	Teddy Roosevelt inaugurated as president	
1901	Vacuum cleaner invented	
1901	Wright brothers test flight at Kitty Hawk	
1902	Teddy Bears marketed after President Teddy Roosevelt's bear hunting incident	
1902	First Harley Davidson motorcycle	
1903	Hand-cranked Victrola invented	
1903	W. E. B. Dubois writes *Souls of Black Folk*	
1904	St. Louis World Fair	
1904	Supreme Court denies African Americans right to vote	
1904	Extension of Chinese Exclusion Act of 1882	
1905	First Yellow Pages	
1905	Nickelodeon (nickel theater) opened in Pittsburgh	
1906	Susan B. Anthony, suffragist, dies before women are granted right to vote	
1906	Fifteen U.S. states have fifteen-mph speed limit	
1906	Food and Drug Act promotes safety in food processing	
1907	First Model T sold for $850	
1907	Ziegfeld Follies	
1908	Plastic invented	
1908	*Christian Science Monitor* founded	
1909	Death of Geronimo in Oklahoma prison	
1909	National Association for the Advancement of Colored People formed	

1910–1919

Social and Historical Timeline		*Client Timeline*
1910	Mexican Revolution	
1910	Boy Scouts and Camp Fire Girls founded	
1911	Amundsen reaches South Pole	
1911	First Hollywood studio makes silent movies	
1911	Andrew Carnegie establishes Carnegie Foundation by donating 90 percent of his fortune	
1911	Architect Frank Lloyd Wright begins construction of Taliesen home and studio	

1912 *Titanic* sinks
1912 X-rays invented
1912 Progressive Party (Teddy Roosevelt) proposes national health insurance
1912 U.S. Public Health Service established
1912 Children's Bureau established
1914 Panama Canal opened
1914 Freud writes *Psychopathology of Everyday Life*
1914 World War I begins
1915 *Lusitania* sinks
1916 National Park Service established
1916 Margaret Sanger opens first birth control clinic
1916 Einstein proposes theory of relativity
1916 Child labor legislation
1917 Russian Revolution and abdication of the czar
1917 Murder of Frank Little, union organizer, in Butte, Montana
1917 Jeannette Rankin first woman in Congress
1917 United States enters World War I
1917 Death of Buffalo Bill Cody
1917 Puerto Rico made a U.S. territory
1918 Carlisle Indian School closed
1918 Supreme Court overrules child labor legislation
1918 Germany accepts Allied Armistice
1918 Supreme Court strikes down minimum wage
1919 League of Nations established
1919 Treaty of Versailles signed
1919 American Legion founded
1919 White Sox scandal
1919 Worldwide influenza epidemic
1919 Nazi Party formed

1920–1929

Social and Historical Timeline *Client Timeline*

1920 Roaring Twenties begins
1920 Harlem Renaissance begins
1920 Prohibition
1920 U.S. population over 100 million
1920 Child Welfare League of America formed
1920 First radio broadcast

1920 Ratification of Nineteenth Amendment grants women the right to vote
1920 Hair bobbing during the sexual revolution
1920 Gandhi leads nonviolent political protests
1921 First Miss America pageant
1921 Fascist Party formed
1922 Mussolini comes to power
1923 Dance marathons
1924 Citizenship Act of 1924 grants Native Americans the right to vote
1924 Immigration Act favors European whites, excludes Asians
1924 Frozen Food invented
1925 Grand Ole Opry begins
1925 John Scopes arrested for teaching evolution
1925 Ku Klux Klan at peak 5 million members
1926 Greyhound Bus Company established
1927 Charles Lindbergh flies solo across Atlantic Ocean to Paris
1929 Talking movies replace silent movies
1929 Stock market crash

1930–1939

Social and Historical Timeline *Client Timeline*

1930 Sliced bread invented
1930 Al Capone is Public Enemy #1
1930 Great Depression begins
1930 Dust Bowl era begins
1930 Veterans Administration established
1931 "Star Spangled Banner" adopted as national anthem
1931 Penicillin first used
1931 Television
1931 Empire State Building opens
1932 Federal Economic Act
1932 Civilian Conservation Corps established
1932 Vaudeville no longer most popular form of entertainment
1933 New Deal under President Franklin Roosevelt
1933 Hitler comes to power in Germany

1933 Tennessee Valley Authority created

1933 Emergency Farm Mortgage Act and Farm Relief Act

1935 Social Security Act passed

1935 Work Projects Association established

1935 National Recovery Act

1935 Big Band era begins

1935 Alcoholics Anonymous formed

1936 Amtrak begins

1937 Nylon stockings invented

1937 Hindenburg burned

1938 Amelia Earhart's plane disappears over the Pacific

1938 Fair Labor Standards Act sets minimum wage at $.25/hour

1939 World War II begins

1940–1949

Social and Historical Timeline *Client Timeline*

1941 Regular television broadcasting begins

1941 Germans invade Russia

1941 Josef Stalin names himself head of the Soviet Union

1941 Japan attacks Pearl Harbor

1941 Jeannette Rankin returns to Congress

1941 USO founded

1941 Manhattan Project authorized to secretly build atomic bomb

1942 U.S. rationing began

1942 Japanese Americans relocated

1942 Planned Parenthood Federation formed

1942 First atomic chain triggered

1944 D-Day invasion of France

1944 GI Bill

1945 Truman orders bombing of Hiroshima

1945 United Nations established

1945 President Franklin Roosevelt dies

1945 Nuremberg trials begin

1945 Trial of Adolf Eichmann, Nazi war criminal

1945 Liberation of Auschwitz concentration camp by Russian Red Army

1946 First computer invented

1946 Baby boom begins
1946 Hill Burton Act supports health care
1946 National school lunch program
1947 Jackie Robinson first black man in major league baseball
1947 Marshall Plan for Europe's reconstruction
1948 State of Israel formed
1949 Margaret Chase Smith first woman to be elected to both houses of Congress
1949 Republic of China established by Chairman Mao

1950–1959

Social and Historical Timeline		*Client Timeline*
1950	Korean War	
1950	Senator Joseph McCarthy's campaign against communism	
1950	Northern migration of African Americans	
1950	Psychotropic drugs	
1950	United States enters Korean War	
1950	First copy machine	
1950	Aid to Families with Dependent Children	
1952	Mr. Potato Head invented	
1953	Korean War ends	
1953	Department of Health, Education and Welfare	
1953	First issue of *Playboy* printed	
1954	Desegregation of schools	
1954	First transistor radio	
1954	Vocational Rehabilitation Act	
1954	"Under God" added to Pledge of Allegiance	
1955	Women earn $.63 for every dollar men earn in the United States	
1955	Disneyland opens	
1955	AFL-CIO formed	
1955	National Association of Social Workers formed	
1955	Montgomery bus boycott	
1955	Polio vaccine invented by Dr. Jonas Salk	
1957	Space Wars begin with Russian launching of *Sputnik*	
1957	Hula hoop invented	
1957	*American Bandstand* goes national	
1958	Nikita Kruschev becomes Russian president	
1959	Barbie dolls	

1960–1969

Social and Historical Timeline		*Client Timeline*
1960	Birth control pill approved	
1960	First televised presidential debate (Nixon and Kennedy)	
1960	Astroturf	
1960	Women of color earn $.42 for every dollar men earn in United States	
1961	Berlin Wall built	
1961	Peace Corps established	
1961	First members of Generation X born	
1961	Cuban Missile Crisis	
1961	U.S. military buildup in Vietnam	
1961	Astronaut Alan Shepard launched into space	
1962	National Farm Workers Union established by Cesar Chavez	
1962	Astronaut John Glenn becomes first to orbit moon	
1962	Vatican II begins	
1963	Martin Luther King delivers "I Have a Dream" speech	
1963	Equal Pay for Equal Work Bill passed	
1963	President John Kennedy assassinated	
1963	Beatles invade United States	
1963	Community Mental Health Centers Act and deinstitutionalization	
1963	Surgeon General's warning on health hazards related to smoking	
1964	Food Stamp Act	
1964	Battered child syndrome identified	
1964	Billy Mills, part Sioux Indian, wins 10,000-meter gold medal in Tokyo Olympics	
1964	VISTA established	
1964	Head Start established	
1964	Poverty line set	
1964	Civil Rights Act passed	
1964	President Lyndon Johnson's War on Poverty	
1965	Miniskirts	
1965	Medicare	
1965	Medicaid	
1965	Older Americans Act	
1966	National Organization for Women founded	
1967	First handheld calculators	

1967	Race riots in Watts
1968	First heart transplant performed
1968	Oil and gas discovered on Alaska North Slope
1968	Shirley Chisholm first black woman elected to Congress
1968	Martin Luther King assassinated
1968	First national Women's Liberation Conference
1969	*Apollo* lands on the moon
1969	Woodstock
1969	Gay rights movement begins
1969	California becomes first state to adopt no-fault divorce laws

1970–1979

Social and Historical Timeline		*Client Timeline*
1970	First Earth Day	
1970	Native American Indian Women's Association formed	
1970	Kent State University students killed by National Guardsmen	
1970	Telephone booth stuffing	
1970	Occupational Safety and Health Act	
1972	Mark Spitz wins seven Olympic gold medals	
1972	First battered women's shelter in United States opens	
1972	Supplemental Security Income established	
1972	Strategic Arms Limitation Treaty signed	
1972	Israeli athletes murdered at Munich Olympics by Palestinian extremists	
1972	*Ms.* magazine founded	
1972	Republicans break into Democratic National Committee headquarters in Watergate Hotel	
1973	Earned income tax credit for individuals	
1973	Work Incentive Program	
1973	American Indian Movement occupation at Wounded Knee	
1973	*Roe v. Wade* abortion decision	
1973	Health Maintenance Organization Act	
1974	Hank Aaron breaks Babe Ruth's home-run record	
1974	Child Abuse and Neglect Treatment Act	
1974	Women's Educational Equity Act passed	
1974	Juvenile Justice and Delinquency Prevention Act	
1974	President Richard Nixon resigns	

1975 Human Rights Pact signed in Helsinki, Finland
1975 Fall of Saigon, South Vietnam
1975 Education for All Handicapped Children Act
1975 Indian Self-Determination Act
1976 United Nation's Decade for Women begins
1976 Title IX of Education Amendments enacted
1976 Inaugural flight of the Concorde
1976 Disco era begins
1977 Montana senator Mike Mansfield appointed ambassador to Japan
1977 Elvis Presley dies
1978 First test tube baby
1978 Sundance Film Festival begins
1978 Indian Child Welfare Act
1978 Pope John Paul selected first non-Italian pope
1979 Shah leaves Iran
1979 Margaret Thatcher elected British prime minister

1980–1989

Social and Historical Timeline — *Client Timeline*

1980 Debut of CNN
1980 Refugee Act allows refugees to receive health and social services
1980 Reaganomics
1980 Omnibus Budget Reconciliation Act brings social program cuts and block grants
1980 Adoption Assistance and Child Welfare Reform Act
1981 AIDS identified
1981 Rubik's cube popular
1981 President Ronald Reagan shot
1981 Pope John Paul shot
1981 Prince Charles marries Diana Spencer
1981 Economic recession
1983 Sandra Day O'Connor confirmed first female Supreme Court justice
1981 Major league baseball strike
1981 Equal Rights Amendment fails
1982 First mechanical heart
1983 Sally Ride first woman astronaut in space
1985 Wilma ManKiller first woman installed chief of a Native American tribe (Cherokee)

1986	Space Shuttle Challenger explodes
1986	U.S. farm crisis
1986	$2 trillion U.S. national debt
1986	Chernobyl nuclear disaster
1986	Iran-Contra scandal broke
1987	First U.S. $1 trillion budget deficit
1987	Exxon oil spill in Valdez, Alaska
1987	McKinney Homeless Assistance Act
1988	Prozac
1988	Family Support Act
1989	Internet
1989	Fall of Berlin Wall
1989	Supreme Court gives states right to regulate abortion

1990–1999

Social and Historical Timeline		*Client Timeline*
1990	Hubble telescope	
1990	Gulf War	
1990	Americans with Disabilities Act	
1991	Fall of the Soviet Union	
1991	World Wide Web invented	
1991	Rodney King beating	
1991	Microsoft Windows 3.0 introduced	
1993	Apartheid ends in South Africa	
1993	Beanie babies	
1993	Family Medical Leave Act	
1993	Native American Free Exercise of Religion Act passed	
1993	North American Free Trade Act	
1993	United States, Russia, England sign Strategic Arms Reduction Treaty	
1993	World Trade Center bombing	
1993	Branch Davidians killed at Waco	
1993	Great Midwest flood	
1993	*Cheers* ends	
1994	Gender Equity in Education Act	
1994	Republican Contract with America	
1995	Violence Against Women Act	
1995	Nelson Mandela elected president of South Africa	
1995	Oklahoma City bombing	
1995	O. J. Simpson trial	

1996	Personal Responsibility and Work Opportunities Act
1996	Taliban captures Kabul
1997	Cloning of Dolly the sheep
1997	Madeline Albright first female secretary of state
1997	Fen-phen diet drug found to be damaging
1998	President William Clinton impeachment trial
1998	Dallas Diocese Catholic sex abuse scandal
1998	Murder of Matthew Shepard
1999	Y2K millennium bug scare
1999	Columbine school shooting

4

Spitituality and Aging

Vicki Murdock

Pretest/Posttest on Spirituality and Aging

1. T or F The First Amendment prohibits Americans from addressing religion in the workplace.
2. T or F Studies as to whether we increase, decrease, or maintain our religious and spiritual beliefs and behaviors as we age are currently inconclusive.
3. T or F The aging population is projected to be about double what it currently is by 2030.
4. T or F It is appropriate to have a discussion about client/patient spirituality only when the client/patient brings up the topic.
5. T or F Empirical research cannot measure human spiritual experience.
6. T or F The elderly are the only people who can integrate across the life span.
7. T or F Helping professionals receive adequate preparation on the topic of addressing client spirituality in their professional education.
8. T or F A diversity-oriented definition of spirituality includes the atheist, the humanist, and the religious believer.
9. T or F Asking about client/patient spirituality may elicit stories of positive and negative spiritual experiences.
10. T or F Over 90 percent of adults in a recent study reported that they had never been asked about their spiritual beliefs by their healthcare professional.
11. T or F Client/patient spirituality should be assessed only in an individual session in order to ensure confidentiality and privacy.
12. T or F All people are spiritual, if the definition of spiritual is inclusive.
13. T or F Asking about childhood religious/spiritual beliefs and behaviors is too time consuming to be effective practice.

14. T or F The majority of patients want their health-care professionals to ask them about their spiritual beliefs.
15. T or F Late-life and end-of-life issues are frightening topics for many clients/patients and professionals.
16. T or F Asking about client/patient religion and spirituality may provide social support intervention opportunities.
17. T or F It is appropriate to use an approach that encourages workers and clients to see all people as the same.
18. T or F Religion includes a community component.

Answers to Pretest/Posttest on Spirituality and Aging

1. F The First Amendment prohibits Americans from addressing religion in the workplace.
2. T Studies as to whether we increase, decrease, or maintain our religious and spiritual beliefs and behaviors as we age are currently inconclusive.
3. T The aging population is projected to about double by 2030.
4. F It is appropriate to have a discussion about client/patient spirituality only when the client/patient brings up the topic.
5. F Empirical research cannot measure human spiritual experience.
6. T The elderly are the only people who can integrate across the life span.
7. F Helping professionals receive adequate preparation on the topic of addressing client spirituality in their professional education.
8. T A diversity-oriented definition of spirituality includes the atheist, the humanist, and the religious believer.
9. T Asking about client/patient spirituality may elicit stories of positive and negative spiritual experiences.
10. T Over 90 percent of adults in a recent study reported that they had never been asked about their spiritual beliefs by their health-care professional.
11. F Client/patient spirituality should be assessed only in an individual session in order to ensure confidentiality and privacy.
12. T All people are spiritual, if the definition of spiritual is inclusive.
13. F Asking about childhood religious/spiritual beliefs and behaviors is too time consuming to be effective practice.
14. T The majority of patients want their health-care professionals to ask them about their spiritual beliefs.
15. T Late-life and end-of-life issues are frightening topics for many clients/patients and professionals.
16. T Asking about client/patient religion and spirituality may provide social support intervention opportunities.
17. F It is appropriate to use an approach that encourages workers and clients to see all people as the same.
18. T Religion includes a community component.

FRAMEWORK FOR SPIRITUAL ASSESSMENT

Initial Narrative Framework

1. Describe the religious/spiritual tradition with which you grew up. How did your family express its spiritual beliefs? How important was spirituality to your family? To your extended family?
2. What sort of personal experiences (practices) during your years at home stand out to you now? What made these experiences special? How have they informed your later life?
3. How have you changed or matured as a result of those experiences? How would you describe your current spiritual or religious orientation? Is your spirituality a personal strength? If so, how?

Interpretive Anthropological Framework

1. Affect: What aspects of your spiritual life give you pleasure? What role does your spirituality play in your ability to handle life's sorrows? Enhance life's joys? Cope with life's pain? How does your spirituality give you hope for the future? What do you wish to accomplish in the future?
2. Behavior: Are there particular spiritual rituals or practices that help you deal with life's obstacles? What is your level of involvement in faith-based communities? How are they supportive? Are there spiritually encouraging individuals with whom you maintain contact?
3. Cognition: What are your current religious/spiritual beliefs? What are they based on? What beliefs do you find particularly meaningful? What does your faith say about personal trials? How does this belief help you overcome obstacles? How do your beliefs affect your health practices?
4. Communion: Describe your relationship with the Ultimate. What has been your experience of the Ultimate? How does the Ultimate communicate with you? How have these experiences encouraged you? Have you experienced times of deep spiritual intimacy? How does your relationship help you face life challenges? How would the Ultimate describe you?
5. Conscience: How do you determine right and wrong? What are your key values? How does your spirituality help you deal with guilt (sin)? What role does forgiveness play in your life?
6. Intuition: To what extent do you experience intuitive hunches (flashes of creative insight, premonitions, spiritual insight)? Have these insights been a strength in your life? If so, how?

SPIRITUAL ASSESSMENT

1. How would you describe your philosophy of life? Of illness? How satisfactory is this philosophy to you now?
2. How do you express you spirituality? What kinds of practices enhance your spirituality?
3. How do you understand hope? What do you hope for?
4. What helps you the most when you feel afraid or need special help?
5. What is especially meaningful to you now? For what do you live? What is most important to you now?
6. How has being sick made any difference in what or how you believe?
7. What do death, being sick, suffering, and pain mean to you?
8. How do you handle feelings such as anger, doubt, resentment, guilt, bitterness, and depression? How does your spirituality influence how you respond to such feelings? Do you want to receive spiritual support to deal with such feelings or thoughts about them?
9. Where do you get the love, courage, strength, hope, and peace that you need?

Questions that use semi-religious language:

1. How is your faith helping or not helping you with your illness?
2. How do you experience God or any other spiritual being(s) to which you relate? (For example, is God loving? If so, in what way?)
3. Where is God for you now? Where is God for you in this experience?
4. How do your spiritual beliefs or your beliefs about the world influence how you respond to your illness? How does your illness influence your spiritual beliefs or your beliefs about the world?

SPIRITUAL/RELIGIOUS HISTORY FORM

F: Do you have a faith or religion that is important to you? Tell me about it.

A: How do your beliefs apply to your health?
Holidays
Fasting
Diet (e.g., caffeine, alcohol)
Lifestyle (e.g., smoking, drugs)
Restrictions (e.g., use of blood products)

I: Are you involved in a faith community, church, or synagogue?
What denomination? Is your faith community a source of support for you? Do you use your pastor or others for counseling?

T: How do your beliefs affect your health-care treatment?

H: How can I help with your spiritual concerns?
Would you like to speak with a chaplain, prayer team, minister, or counselor?

FICA SPIRITUAL ASSESSMENT TOOL

F:	Faith	What is your faith tradition?
I:	Important	How important is your faith to you?
C:	Church	What is your church or community of faith?
A:	Apply/Address	How do your religious and spiritual beliefs apply to your health? How might we address your spiritual needs?

SPIRITUAL SELF-ASSESSMENT

Mark your feelings anywhere along the continuum.

Loneliness . . . . Community

Anxiety/Fear . . . . Peace

Guilt . . . . Forgiveness

Anger/Hostility . . . . Resolution

Meaninglessness . . . . Hope

Grief . . . . Consolation

THE HOPE APPROACH TO SPIRITUAL ASSESSMENT

H: Hope, meaning, comfort, strength, peace, love, and connection
What is there in your life that gives you internal support?
What are your sources of hope, strength, comfort, and peace?
What do you hold on to during difficult times?
What sustains you and keeps you going?
Are religious or spiritual beliefs a comfort in dealing with life's ups and downs? (If so, go on to O and P; if not, ask, Was it ever? What changed?)

O: Organized religion
Do you consider yourself part of an organized religion?
How important is this to you?
What aspects of your religion are helpful and not so helpful to you?
Are you part of a religious or spiritual community? Does it help you? How?

P: Personal spirituality/practices

Do you have personal spiritual beliefs that are independent of organized religion? What are they? Do you believe in God? What kind of relationship do you have with God?

What aspects of your spirituality or spiritual practice do you find most helpful (e.g., prayer, meditation, reading scripture, attending religious services, listening to music, hiking, communing with nature)?

E: Effects on medical care and end-of-life issues

Has being sick (or your current situation) affected your ability to do the things that usually help you spiritually (or has your situation affected your relationship with God)?

Is there anything I can do to help you access the resources that usually help you?

Are you worried about any conflicts between your beliefs and your medical situation/care/decisions?

Would it be helpful for you to speak to a chaplain, community spiritual leader, or counselor?

Are there any specific practice or restrictions I should know about in providing care to you?

If the patient is dying: How do your beliefs affect the kind of care you would like me to provide over the next days?

The Spiritual Experience Index

Circle the response that most closely corresponds to how you feel about each statement. SD = strongly disagree; D = disagree; SWD = somewhat disagree; SWA = somewhat agree; A = agree; SA = strongly agree

	Statement						
1.	I often feel close to a power greater than myself.	SD	D	SWD	SWA	A	SA
2.	I often feel that I have little control over what happens to me.	SD	D	SWD	SWA	A	SA
3.	My faith gives my life meaning and purpose.	SD	D	SWD	SWA	A	SA
4.	My faith is a way of life.	SD	D	SWD	SWA	A	SA
5.	Ideas from faiths different from my own may increase my understanding of spiritual truth.	SD	D	SWD	SWA	A	SA
6.	One should not marry someone of a different faith.	SD	D	SWD	SWA	A	SA
7.	My faith is an important part of my individual identity.	SD	D	SWD	SWA	A	SA
8.	My faith helps me to confront tragedy and suffering.	SD	D	SWD	SWA	A	SA
9.	My faith is often a deeply emotional experience.	SD	D	SWD	SWA	A	SA
10.	It is difficult for me to form a clear, concrete image of God.	SD	D	SWD	SWA	A	SA
11.	I believe that there is only one true faith.	SD	D	SWD	SWA	A	SA
12.	It is important that I follow the religious beliefs of my parents.	SD	D	SWD	SWA	A	SA
13.	Learning about different faiths is an important part of my spiritual development.	SD	D	SWD	SWA	A	SA
14.	I often think about issues concerning my faith.	SD	D	SWD	SWA	A	SA
15.	If my faith is strong enough, I will not experience doubt.	SD	D	SWD	SWA	A	SA
16.	Obedience to religious doctrine is the most important aspect of my faith.	SD	D	SWD	SWA	A	SA

17.	My relationship with God is experienced as unconditional love.	SD	D	SWD	SWA	A	SA
18.	My spiritual beliefs change as I encounter new ideas and experiences.	SD	D	SWD	SWA	A	SA
19.	I am sometimes uncertain about the best way to resolve a moral conflict.	SD	D	SWD	SWA	A	SA
20.	I often fear God's punishment.	SD	D	SWD	SWA	A	SA
21.	Although I sometimes fall short of my spiritual ideals, I am still basically a good and worthwhile person.	SD	D	SWD	SWA	A	SA
22.	A primary purpose of prayer is to avoid personal tragedy.	SD	D	SWD	SWA	A	SA
23.	I can experience spiritual doubts and still remain committed to my faith.	SD	D	SWD	SWA	A	SA
24.	I believe that the world is basically good.	SD	D	SWD	SWA	A	SA
25.	My faith enables me to experience forgiveness when I act against my moral conscience.	SD	D	SWD	SWA	A	SA
26.	It is important that my spiritual beliefs conform with those those of the people closest to me.	SD	D	SWD	SWA	A	SA
27.	Persons of different faiths share a common spiritual bond.	SD	D	SWD	SWA	A	SA
28.	I gain spiritual strength by trusting in a higher power.	SD	D	SWD	SWA	A	SA
29.	There is usually only one right solution to any moral dilemma.	SD	D	SWD	SWA	A	SA
30.	I make a conscious effort to live in accordance with my spiritual values.	SD	D	SWD	SWA	A	SA
31.	I feel a strong spiritual bond with all humankind	SD	D	SWD	SWA	A	SA
32.	My faith is a private experience that I rarely, if ever, share with others.	SD	D	SWD	SWA	A	SA
33.	Sharing my faith with others is important for my spiritual growth.	SD	D	SWD	SWA	A	SA
34.	I never challenge the teachings of my faith.	SD	D	SWD	SWA	A	SA

35.	I believe that the world is basically evil.	SD	D	SWD	SWA	A	SA
36.	Religious scriptures are best interpreted as symbolic attempts to convey ultimate truths.	SD	D	SWD	SWA	A	SA
37.	My faith guides my whole approach to life.	SD	D	SWD	SWA	A	SA
38.	Improving the human community is an important spiritual goal.	SD	D	SWD	SWA	A	SA

THE SPIRITUAL HISTORY

S: Spiritual belief system
What is your formal religious affiliation?
Name or describe your spiritual belief system.

P: Personal spirituality
Describe the beliefs and practices of your religion or spiritual system that you personally accept.
Describe the beliefs or practices you do not accept.
Do you accept or believe in [specific tenet or practice]?
What does your spirituality/religion mean to you?
What is the importance of your spirituality/religion in daily life?

I: Integration with a spiritual community
Do you belong to any spiritual or religious group or community?
What is your position or role?
Is it a source of support? In what ways?
Does or could this group provide help in dealing with health issues?

R: Ritualized practice and restrictions
Are there specific practices that you carry out as part of your religion/spirituality (e.g., prayer, meditation)?
Are there certain lifestyle activities or practices that your religion/spirituality encourages or forbids? Do you comply?
What significance do these practices and restrictions have to you?
Are there elements of medical care that you refuse to receive on the basis of religious/spiritual grounds?

I: Implications
What aspects of your religion/spirituality would you like me to keep in mind as I care for you?
Would you like to discuss the religious or spiritual implications of your care?
What knowledge or understanding would strengthen our relationship as provider and patient?

Do you feel there are there any barriers to our relationship based on religious or spiritual issues?

T: Terminal events planning

As we plan for your care near the end of life, how does your faith affect your decisions?

Are there particular aspects of care that you wish to forgo or have withheld because of your faith?

REFERENCES

Anandarajah, G., & Hight, E. (2001). Spirituality and medical practice: Using the HOPE questions as a practical tool for spiritual assessment. *American Family Physician, 63,* 81–89. Retrieved from http://www.aafp.org/afp/20010101/81.html

Blanchard, J. (2002, January/February). Coping with illness: Your spiritual journey. *Association of Professional Chaplains Newsletter.*

Dudley, J. R., Smith, C., & Millison, M. B. (1995). Unfinished business: Assessing the spiritual needs of hospice clients. *American Journal of Hospice and Palliative Care, 12*(2), 30–37.

Genia, V. (1991). The spiritual experience index: A measure of spiritual maturity. *Journal of Religion and Health, 30*(4), 337–347.

Hodge, D. R. (2001). Spiritual assessment: A review of major qualitative methods and a new framework for assessing spirituality. *Social Work, 46*(3), 203–214.

King, D. E. (2000). *Faith, spirituality, and medicine: Toward the making of the healing practitioner.* New York: Haworth Pastoral Press.

Maugans, T. A. (1996). The SPIRITual history. *Archives of Family Medicine, 5*(8), 439.

Puchalski, C. M. (1999). Taking a spiritual history: FICA. *Spirituality and Medicine Connection, 3*(1), 1.

Part Three

Self-Reflective Exercises

5

Psychosocial Aspects of Chronic and Terminal Illness

Taking Care of Our Patients and Ourselves

Hillel Bodek

This questionnaire has three purposes: (1) to help health-care professionals begin to think about psychosocial-spiritual issues relating to illness, death, and dying; (2) to help health-care professionals begin to think about and gain insight and self-awareness into how they deal with these issues personally, which will affect how they deal with these issues with chronically and terminally ill individuals and their families; (3) to help develop teaching materials about issues of spirituality in relation to palliative and end-of-life care.

This questionnaire is confidential. Your name is not requested and should not be placed on it.

Issues relating to illness, death, dying, and spirituality are sensitive ones. If there are any particular questions you find you are uncomfortable responding to, do not feel you must answer them.

List three things that give the most meaning to your life.

1. ____
2. ____
3. ____

List three activities that you enjoy.

1. ____
2. ____
3. ____

List three goals, hopes, dreams, or aspirations you have.

1. ______________________________

2. ______________________________

3. ______________________________

List three things that people fear most about chronic illness.

1. ______________________________

2. ______________________________

3. ______________________________

List three things that people fear most about death.

1. ______________________________

2. ______________________________

3. ______________________________

List three reactions/behaviors that people have or exhibit in response to learning that they have a terminal illness.

1. ______________________________

2. ______________________________

3. ______________________________

List three losses that people may experience during their lifetime, and rate them from most to least serious.

1. ______________________________

2. ______________________________

3. ______________________________

List your three greatest concerns about working with chronically/terminally ill patients and their families.

1. ______________________________

2. ______________________________

3. ______________________________

List three things that might prevent you from providing effective palliative and end-of-life care.

1. ______________________________

2. ______________________________

3. ______________________________

Consider for a moment the most wonderful death you can imagine for yourself. It doesn't have to be realistic; it can be quite fantastic. You might not have thought about this before. Give it your best shot. The only caveat is that you must die. There is no way out. Where are you? Who is with you? What are you doing? Are you experiencing any physical or emotional symptoms? How long have you known you are dying?

____

____

____

____

____

____

____

____

____

____

What three events/experiences have shaped your life the most?

1. ______________________________

2. ______________________________

3. ______________________________

What are the three things that motivate you the most?

1. ______________________________

2. ______________________________

3. ______________________________

Which three things give the most meaning to your life?

1. ____
2. ____
3. ____

What do you consider the three core values that you use to guide your life?

1. ____
2. ____
3. ____

What are the three happiest events in your life?

1. ____
2. ____
3. ____

What are the three most painful/saddest events in your life?

1. ____
2. ____
3. ____

List three things you most want to accomplish during your lifetime.

1. ____
2. ____
3. ____

What are the three biggest regrets in your life?

1. ____
2. ____
3. ____

What three things do you view as your greatest accomplishments?

1. ____
2. ____
3. ____

If you had to live your life up to this point all over again, what three things would you do differently?

1. ____

2. ____

3. ____

If you had six months to live, what five things would you want to do during that time?

1. ____

2. ____

3. ____

4. ____

5. ____

If you died today, what do you feel are the three most important things you would leave incomplete or unaccomplished?

1. ____

2. ____

3. ____

What do you want your legacy to be after you die?

1. ____

2. ____

3. ____

List three ways your profession has affected your life.

1. ____

2. ____

3. ____

What would you do if you left your profession?

1. ____

2. ____

3. ____

How would leaving your health-care profession affect your life?

1. ______________________________

2. ______________________________

3. ______________________________

If, when, and under what conditions would you like to retire?

____

____

What three things do you most want to do when you retire?

1. ______________________________

2. ______________________________

3. ______________________________

If you learned that you were terminally ill and had only a few months to live, what three things would you fear most about your impending death?

1. ______________________________

2. ______________________________

3. ______________________________

If you learned that you had a chronic illness that would be fatal within two years, what are the four most important things you would want your physician/nurse/social worker to do for you during the period of your illness?

1. ______________________________

2. ______________________________

3. ______________________________

4. ______________________________

If you learned that you had a chronic illness that would be fatal within two years, what are the four most important things you would want your chaplain to do for you during the the period of your illness?

1. ______________________________

2. ______________________________

3. ______________________________

4. ______________________________

If you had a chronic illness and knew that you were now in the final days of your life, what are the four most important things you would want your physician/nurse/social worker to do for you during these final days?

1. ______________________________

2. ______________________________

3. ______________________________

4. ______________________________

If you had a chronic illness and knew that you were now in the final days of your life, what are the four most important things you would want your chaplain to do for you during these final days?

1. ______________________________

2. ______________________________

3. ______________________________

4. ______________________________

6

Some Death/Dying/Loss Activities for the Classroom

Vicki Murdock

Bring in an object that represents a significant loss; discuss the feelings of loss still present even after many years.

Write or talk about your first childhood experience with death: at what age did it occur, how do you remember it, who died, and what was said to you? (Klick, 1999). How do various cultures differ in approaching the topic of death with children?

Write your own obituary; discuss the process of writing it, as well as the content, in small groups. Alternatively, plan your funeral and discuss the thoughts and feelings that come up for you around this activity (Cohen, 2002).

Debate issues in mental health and aging: the right to die, the right to refuse medical treatment, who decides competence, late-life learning, autonomy versus safety, the right to self-neglect, disengagement theory/activity theory, genetic screening, late-life wisdom/creativity, meaning of life in a youth-oriented culture, mandatory or "encouraged" retirement, older adult suicide, lifesaving medical care for people with Alzheimer's, the purpose and benefits of mental health therapy with the elderly. This activity, like any debate, must be set up carefully so that everyone is aware that the debaters take a stand that is not necessarily their own personal belief.

Complete a living will for yourself (not to be signed or witnessed within the context of this activity); write a reflection paper on your thoughts and feelings after completing the exercise (Haulotte & Kretszchmar, 2001). This activity can engender lots of discussion; hopefully, exposure to advance directives will spur the student to complete official forms and encourage others to do so, too.

Imagine you have just received a letter from an old friend expressing thoughts in favor of suicide. Write a letter to the friend giving your reasons for agreeing or disagreeing with the conclusions he or she has reached (Moody, 1998).

This is another example of an activity that requires the preparation of a safe environment for students to share.

Write down five things you highly value. One by one, cross off the items, allowing time to experience, in imagination only, the sense of loss and despair that accompanies the loss of things of great value. Or list roles and then take them away (Morano, 2002). This activity takes only moments but produces strong feelings and interesting discussion.

Take a longevity test (available at http://www.nmfn.com/tn/learnctr-life events-longevity or www.livingto100.com). Discuss or write about your feelings regarding the questions asked and the results.

Create a timeline of losses; with a partner, discuss feelings engendered and potential for this graphic intervention to normalize the grieving of loss. This activity stimulates great variety in how the graphic is drawn, from straight lines to spirals and symbols.

Complete a life review or spiritual history on yourself in with another student or with an older adult (Hodge, 2001). Create a keepsake by crafting a product from the interview.

Create a suicide contract. With a partner, check it for thoroughness and for its effect on both worker and client; process your feelings around preparing and writing this document and imagining its use with a client. Or use the Suicidal Ideation treatment plan (Frazer & Jongsma, 1999).

Personal History of Losses

Use questions in interview form or complete on paper

1. The first death I can remember was the death of
2. I was age
3. The feelings I remember I had at the time were
4. The first funeral, wake, or memorial service I ever attended was for
5. I was age
6. The thing I most remember about that experience is
7. My most recent loss from death was
8. I coped with this loss by
9. The most difficult death for me was the death of
10. It was difficult because
11. Of the important people in my life who are now living, the most difficult death for me would be the death of
12. It would be the most difficult because
13. My primary style of coping with loss is
14. I know my own grief is resolved when
15. It is appropriate to share my own experiences with others as a way to help them when

REFERENCES

Cohen, H. L. (2002). Social work with older adults. In N. P. Kropf & C. J. Tompkins (Eds.), *Teaching aging: Syllabi, resources, and infusion materials for the social work curriculum* (pp. 57–67). Alexandria, VA: Council on Social Work Education.

Frazer, D. W., & Jongsma, A. E. (1999). *The older adult psychotherapy treatment planner.* New York: John Wiley and Sons.

Haulotte, S. M., & Kretzschmar, J. A. (2001). *Case scenarios for teaching and learning social work practice.* Alexandria, VA: Council on Social Work Education.

Hodge, D. (2001). Spiritual assessment: A review of major qualitative methods and a new framework for assessing spirituality. *Social Work, 46*(3), 203–214.

Klick, A. (1999). Death and bereavement. In V. Richardson (Ed.), *Teaching gerontological social work: A compendium of model syllabi* (pp. 71–79). Alexandria, VA: Council on Social Work Education.

Moody, H. R. (1998). *Aging: Concepts and controversies* (3rd ed.). Thousand Oaks, CA: Pine Forge Press.

Morano, C. (2002). Membership exercise. In N. P. Kropf & C. J. Tompkins (Eds.), *Teaching aging: Syllabi, resources, and infusion materials for the social work curriculum* (pp. 160–165). Alexandria, VA: Council on Social Work Education.

Worden, J. W. (2002). *Grief counseling and grief therapy: A handbook for the mental health practitioner* (3rd ed.). New York: Springer.

Part Four

Assignments

7

Loss, Grief, and Social Work Interventions

Cynthia Forrest

THEORY CRITIQUE

What is the social work concern related to practice with people facing life-threatening illnesses that you are interested in exploring? Examples are examining how people facing life-threatening illnesses experience and move through the progressive losses associated with illness, how children experience grief, how agencies develop and respond to care needs, or the implications of public policies' influence on quality and quantity of care. (Don't limit yourself—be creative.)

Explain why you chose this concern. Provide evidence (what does the literature say?) of how this concern affects people's lives, agency functioning, and other professional service provision.

Identify one social work theory you will be critiquing. Explain the primary principles of practice this theory/perspective uses. Use this theory as the framework to explore the matter you are concerned with, providing details of how this theory explains the concern you are discussing. This is the "rubber meets the road" piece. In other words, discuss issues related to your concern using the lens of this theory.

Provide a detailed critique of the theory's relevance to the matter you are concerned with. Discuss the theory's strengths in explaining the matter from a social work perspective. Discuss the theory's limitations in explaining the matter from a social work perspective. Is this theory better suited for explaining direct practice issues, large systems issues, or both? Justify your response.

REFLECTIVE PAPER 1

Identify three major themes and areas of content discussed in the readings and in class. Discuss the two major areas that made the greatest impression on you. Explain your response. How will this information help you in your role as a social worker?

Based on the hopes, wishes, and expectations you identified on the first day of class, how do you plan on using this course to achieve your goals? It is likely that based on your personal experiences with loss, grief, and death, you will have an emotional response to some of the content discussed in this course. How do you plan on taking care of yourself over the course of the semester?

REFLECTIVE PAPER 2

From the readings and discussions in class, identify two major contemporary models of professional caregiving and describe how they influence the care of people facing end-of-life matters. Discuss the two major areas in the reading that made the greatest impression on you. Explain your response. How will this information help you understand some of the strengths and struggles experienced by your mentor and his or her family?

In thinking about your own quality-of-life concerns, what do you consider most important and least important to feeling that your life is worth living? How might your values influence or affect your work with others who are facing life-threatening illnesses?

REFLECTIVE PAPER 3

Describe two theories of grief. Use one of the theories you described to discuss how a person's culture might affect how he or she moves through the model's formula. Discuss how age-related developmental matters might fit into the stages of the second theory you chose. Based on your early interactions with your mentor, identify any healthy and problematic grieving patterns you have witnessed or heard about from the individual or family. Describe these patterns and any effects they have on the family or individual.

How might your own experiences with loss (or lack thereof) influence your ability to understand others' perceptions of loss and the meaning other people attach to experiences of loss?

REFLECTIVE PAPER 4

Discuss the three social work skills you believe are the most critical for enhancing effective communication with individuals and families. From an interdisciplinary team perspective, discuss three ways social work professionals participate in care by providing discipline-specific services.

Describe the communication patterns between your mentor, his or her family, and the health-care professionals providing care. In looking at your own communication style and your understanding of the communication skills needed in social work practice with people and systems dealing with life-threatening or end-of-life matters, what do you see as your greatest strength? What do you see as your greatest struggle? How do you imagine these strengths and struggles might influence your position as a member of an interdisciplinary team?

REFLECTIVE PAPER 5

Discuss two major legal and ethical considerations in social work practice regarding either physician-assisted suicide or euthanasia. What do you see as social work's responsibility in addressing ethical and legal concerns related to end-of-life care and support of choice? What do you understand your mentor's thoughts and wishes for a good death to be? If you haven't discussed this or are not comfortable discussing this with your mentor or his or his family, how would you imagine approaching this issue?

What conditions would need to be present in order for you to experience a good death?

REFLECTIVE PAPER 6

Describe one public policy related to end-of-life care. Describe two ways the policy has affected the development of and/or implementation of services for people facing life-threatening illnesses. What evidence of the impact of this policy do you see in the lives of your mentor and his or her family?

Looking back over the semester, what have been your greatest lessons for professional care? What have been your greatest personal lessons?

MENTORING ASSIGNMENT

Each student will be assigned a mentor for the semester. Mentors will be selected from diverse health-care practice settings. Students will be required to visit their mentor for a minimum of six hours over the course of the semester. This will require several visits, as the student will stay only as long as the mentor wants him or her to stay. Students will visit mentors in their homes or at the location that is most convenient for the mentor. They will spend time talking and, more importantly, listening as their mentors share what it is like to live with a life-threatening illness. Students will be required to complete three assignments related to their experiences with their mentors. Mentors and staff at the support agency will receive copies of the assignments. No identifying information about the mentor will be used in the assignments. Mentors must have a diagnosis of a life-threatening illness and be connected with a health-care provider. Students will not perform any official social work services for or on behalf of their mentors. Should needs arise or become evident, the student will notify the social worker or other medical provider.

Hello.

My name is ______________________ and I am a social worker. I work at __________________. I will be teaching a class this __________________ to help students learn how to be good social workers with people who have a serious illness. One of the best ways that students can learn about being a good social worker is by talking with and listening to people who are living with a serious illness.

You are getting this letter because your social worker or other medical helper thinks you might be interested in working with a student in my class. If you are interested in being a mentor, here is what this would mean:

You will be assigned a student from my class who will visit you and/or your family several times during the semester. The student will travel to your home or a place you choose.

The student will meet with you for at least six hours over the course of this class. Each visit will last only as long as you want the student to stay.

The student will listen to what you have to say about what you think is important for social workers to know about working with someone who has a serious illness. In this way you will be a teacher for the student.

The student will keep all conversations with you private, unless the student learns that you may be thinking of hurting yourself or someone else.

Some of the assignments each student completes for this class will be based on what he or she is learning from you. Your name will not be used in the assignments. If you like, your student can show you a copy of the assignments.

I am hoping that with your help, students can learn how to be a better social worker to people who have a serious illness. I also hope that being a mentor will be a good experience for you. You may find the extra support you get from having a student to talk to helpful.

If you want more information or if you are interested in volunteering to be a mentor, please call me at _____________, or ask your social worker or medical helper to call me.

Sincerely,

Volunteer Mentor Informed Consent

I agree to volunteer as a mentor for a masters-level student who is enrolled in a social work course on loss, grief, and social work at ________________. This class is for students who are interested in learning how to be better social workers to people living with a serious illness.

I understand that being a mentor means that

- I will be helping a student understand what it is like living with a serious illness by talking about my experiences and feelings.
- The student will travel either to my home or to a place we choose that is comfortable and convenient for me.
- I will spend six hours with my student between ______________ and ______________.
- The student will keep all our conversations private, unless he or she learns that I may be thinking of hurting myself or someone else.
- The student will not be responsible for any social work services on my behalf. If there are concerns about my welfare, he or she will talk with my social worker or other health-care provider in order to get me the help I need.
- The instructor for this course is interested in hearing about my experiences as a mentor and may ask to talk with me about these experiences during and/or at the end of the course.
- Neither my name nor any identifying information about me or my family will be used in any assignments or reports related to this class.
- I can decide to stop being a mentor at any time without consequences from my health-care provider.

I understand that I may benefit from being a mentor. Possible benefits include knowing that I am helping a future social worker learn how to be a better helper to someone living with a life-threatening illness. I may also benefit from the companionship of my student.

I also understand that the possible risks of being a mentor are that I am agreeing to spend six hours with the student and may be asked to talk with the instructor about my experiences as a mentor. This may present an inconvenience to me. Another risk is that in talking with the student, I may experience uncomfortable feelings.

______________________________	______________________________
Print Name	Signature
______________________________	______________________________
Date	Contact Number

8

Care for the Dying

Helen Harris

Critical book review: Write a review (minimum 5 pages) of a book that deals with illness, death and dying, and care of the dying and their families. The book must be preapproved by the professor, and the book review should follow the review format used by the *Journal for Family Ministry*.

Design your own assignment: Design a project that will assist you in achieving the learning objectives of this course. Your project must be approved by the professor. Some options are writing a song, creating an art project or a slide show, and videotaping interviews.

Paper describing church doctrinal positions and procedures for addressing the needs of the dying and their families: Write a paper (minimum 5 pages) that delineates the church or denominational position statement regarding needs and care of the dying and their families, specific church ministries (formal and informal) to the dying and their families, and any training or instruction required by the church or available in the church for ministerial staff working with the dying and their families.

9

Loss and Grief
Individual, Family, and Cultural Perspectives

Barbara Jones

FINAL PAPER OPTION 1: GRIEF AND LOSS ASSESSMENT—CASE ANALYSIS

Goal: To integrate the knowledge and skills gained in this course with work that you are doing in the field. Specifically, you will be utilizing your assessment skills to conduct a grief assessment / loss history with a client.

Process: Identify a client from your current or previous caseload for whom issues of grief and loss are relevant. The loss event does not need to be the presenting problem or reason for referral. However, be sure to select a client whose loss history is already familiar to you or from whom you have the ability to gather additional information. Also remember to protect client confidentiality; however, be careful not to change the client's age significantly if you are working with a child. You may want to share a copy of this assignment with your field instructor. This may enhance his or her ability to help you integrate course material with your field work.

Product: Using the following headings and guidelines, you will create an APA-style paper of fifteen to twenty pages that integrates your learning in this class. Be sure to use critical thinking, cultural humility, and an integration of grief-and-loss theory to prepare a comprehensive case analysis / loss assessment that provides the following information.

1. Field agency: Briefly describe your field agency and your role(s) within the agency (one or two paragraphs).
2. Introduction to the case: Briefly describe your client system (individual, family, or group). Provide first name(s) and age(s) but do not go into the client's history here—save that for section 4. Discuss how long and in what capacity you have worked with this client.

3. Assessment strategies:

   - Describe the strategies and process of conducting a grief assessment/ loss history with this client. Be detailed and include agency strategies for assessment such as intake forms and client history. Also identify your personal/professional strategies such as awareness of verbal and nonverbal communication, setting, and relationship.
   - Identify a standardized instrument or questionnaire that would assist you in assessing grief and loss issues with this client. Include a copy of the instrument and be sure to cite the source. Describe how this instrument or questionnaire would be useful in your work. Discuss potential barriers to the use of the standardized instrument with your client.

4. Client grief assessment / loss history: Write a detailed grief and bereavement assessment / loss history in narrative form (i.e., a psychosocial assessment that could be used as a free-standing document in a case file) that includes the following:

   - Identifying information, referral source, and presenting problem
   - Brief social history
   - A comprehensive grief assessment / loss history as described in the readings and class discussions—this should include previous losses; multiple losses; elements of disenfranchisement; reactions to loss; significance and personal meaning of the loss; and impact of gender, race, culture, and age
   - An assessment summary highlighting your conclusions about the case and integrating the facts of the case to critically reflect and to provide clinical assessment of your client.

5. Evaluation of the assessment process

   - Do you feel that you were able to conduct a comprehensive bereavement assessment / loss history in this case? Describe client-related, worker-related, and situational factors that facilitated and/or inhibited the assessment process.
   - List specific categories or pieces of information that you feel are required for a comprehensive understanding of the case but were not available to you for inclusion in the narrative.

6. Support for your conclusions: Provide support for the conclusions that you have reached in this case. In your discussion, you should:

   - Use course materials and at least two references not listed on the syllabus to link facts from your case to relevant information found in the literature

- Identify grief- and loss-related theoretical/conceptual frameworks that influenced your work with this client. How did the frameworks assist you with the assessment process? How did the frameworks assist you with your assessment conclusions? In your discussion, link components of the frameworks with appropriate illustrations and examples for the case (be specific).

7. Recommendations for intervention: Combine your comprehensive assessment of your client with the various strategies for helping that you learned in this class, and design an initial clinical intervention plan for this client. Support your choice of intervention with information about your client and with readings from the course and the scholarly literature.

FINAL PAPER OPTION 2: INTERVENTION AND EVALUATION

Goal: To design an intervention strategy and evaluation plan based upon clinical practice literature and theory to assist clients in coping with issues of grief and loss; to become familiar with the range of resources available for use with clients experiencing loss

Process: Identify a grief/loss event of interest. It does not have to be related to a client or case from the field. You will be researching a potential intervention strategy and evaluation plan (hypothetical rather than based on an actual case) for use in your social work practice with clients experiencing this type of illness. You will also be identifying potential informational and supportive resources available to your clients.

Product: Using the following headings and guidelines, you will create an APA-style paper of eight to fifteen pages:

1. Loss event and rationale: Identify the loss event that you have selected for this assignment. Use course materials and references from the literature that are not on your syllabus to inform your responses to the following questions:

   - Discuss the importance and relevance of this topic for social work practice. (How common is it? How can social workers make a difference in the lives of those experiencing this grief or loss event? Why is social work a logical discipline to assist clients experiencing this grief or loss event?) Think about the values and philosophies underlying social work practice as well as social work's mission.
   - Based upon the literature (and perhaps your personal or professional experience), list potential consequences of the loss and potential problems that might be faced by a person experiencing this loss event.

- Based upon the literature (and perhaps your personal or professional experience), list potential service- and resource-related needs (consider immediate needs as well as longer-term needs).

2. Potential intervention strategy: Using the practice literature to guide you (at least three to four references that are not on your syllabus and any relevant references from the syllabus), describe an intervention strategy that could be used in session to assist a client dealing with this grief or loss event. Describe the intervention in enough detail that a reader could carry it out. If the reference contains specific instructions for implementing the intervention, include them and any supporting materials (e.g., copy of an exercise, description of a film to be shown) in an appendix.
3. Treatment planning / evaluation strategies: Identify potential goals of the intervention that you proposed in section 2—be sure to stay focused on grief- and loss-related goals. In other words, identify anticipated outcomes of this intervention. How might you and your client monitor the success of the intervention? Briefly describe strategies that you might use for evaluating progress toward these treatment goals. Hints for success on section 3:
    - Remember the criteria that facilitate communication about goals/outcomes—they should be specific, concrete, measurable, observable, and so forth. Beware of goals/outcomes that are vague and not clearly defined.
    - Be sure to consider a range of strategies for monitoring and evaluating progress—draw on what you learned in practice and research courses.
    - Discuss ethical dilemmas that could present themselves in your intervention.
4. Rationale for the intervention strategy: Using references from your syllabus and at least two references from the scholarly literature that are not listed on your syllabus, find support for your intervention strategy. How does this intervention relate to the potential problems and/or treatment goals identified in parts 1 and 3? Be sure to discuss how the proposed intervention and the potential problems and anticipated outcomess of treatment are logically connected. Identify at least one grief-related theoretical framework or practice model from the course readings that informs and/or supports this intervention strategy, and discuss its relevance.
5. Factors influencing implementation of the intervention: Identify and describe factors that could hypothetically influence the implementation and success of this intervention plan. Consider the following:

- Client characteristics, resources, and/or circumstances, including issues of diversity, oppression, and discrimination
- Your personal style, comfort levels, and skills
- Constraints created by agency context, policies, or guidelines

6. Potential referral resources: Consider additional resources that might be useful to a client dealing with this loss event. Create a mini-directory that might serve as a referral resource to address the loss event you have chosen with at least one resource in each of the following categories: (1) a community or national agency or organization—briefly describe the grief or loss-related services they provide, (2) a support group (based in the community or online), and (3) educational materials (books, films, pamphlets, online information). Include enough information about each resource that a client could access it (i.e., copy of the resource or information about how to obtain it; name of contact person and telephone number, Web site address).

10

Selected Aspects of Social Work and Social Welfare

Introductory Seminar in End of Life in Rural Communities

Susan Murty

REFLECTIVE JOURNAL ASSIGNMENTS

You will keep a weekly journal in which you will reflect on your personal perceptions, ideas, and reactions to the class. The journal provides an opportunity for you to reflect on the issues related to the class in ways that can bring about self-awareness and personal insights that may improve your practice. Reflect on what the material means to you as it is presented in the texts, on the Web site, and in class. Address your personal reactions. Did you learn anything about yourself? Note any indication of your own concerns, biases, and stereotypes. Assess personal attitudes related to your own eventual aging and death and the aging and death of people important to you. Comment on how your personal reactions might affect your practice, and how you and others might be able address them. You might answer questions such as:

- What am I learning?
- What insights am I gaining about others, society, and myself?
- How comfortable am I in thinking about my own aging and death?
- How will this experience affect my work with people who are dying and their families? With people who are bereaved?

The journal will be private and will be read by the instructors only. There are no right or wrong things to include; the process of completing the journal will be a personal growth experience that may enhance your practice in end-of-life care and bereavement.

FINAL PAPER

Present a plan for rural community assessment of assets and needs related to end-of-life care, palliative care, and/or bereavement, taking into consideration any diverse rural populations in the community, such as Latinos.

1. Select a rural community that you would like to learn more about.
2. Discuss the ways in which the community is rural. How rural is it in light of some of the characteristics of rural communities we have discussed in class?
3. Gather some data concerning the population of the community, including ethnic diversity, recent immigrants, and percentage of elderly in the population. Use sources on the Web to help you. (Note that census data may only be available for the county rather than for the particular community you have in mind.)
4. Complete an initial rural community assessment to identify assets that might be helpful to the improvement of end-of-life care in this particular community.
    - Gather data from local newspapers, bulletin boards, phone books, and conversations with residents from at least one visit, using methods described by Hardcastle et al. and Murty.
    - Using sources of information such as those listed above, try to determine the boundaries of the community from the point of view of the residents. Do any nearby small towns belong to the community?
    - Identify the formal regional services that include the community in their service areas (for example, the area agency on aging, the nearest hospitals and nursing homes, hospice programs, home health programs, the public health program, the community mental health program).
5. Describe how you could use the information you have gathered to plan a more in-depth assessment of the needs and assets of the community in relation to end-of-life care, palliative care, and bereavement. Identify some community assets that could help you gather more information from the residents about their concerns and their willingness to assist. What methods would you use? Who would you seek out to be your allies and champions? How could you gain their trust? Be very specific and use the information you have gathered in your initial assessment. For example, rather than saying that you will contact the churches in the community, name the churches and tell how you plan to approach them and who you will contact.

WEB ASSIGNMENT

Choose one or more of the following topics: end-of-life care, palliative care, and bereavement services. You will be supplied with a list of Web sites for each topic. Visit at least five Web sites related to the topic(s) you have chosen. Try to identify the organization that sponsors each Web site. What is its mission? What is the goal of the Web site? What is it trying to persuade you of? What does the site want you to do? Write a brief report (1–2 pages) comparing and contrasting the Web sites. Identify your favorite one or two sites, and say why.

11

Grief and Loss

Practice with Individuals and Groups

Jane Roberts

FINAL PAPER

The purpose of this assignment is to gain a theoretical understanding of the issues related to direct practice with individuals and families coping with illness. Please do the following:

1. Select a factor related to grief and loss that is of interest to you.
2. Do library research to learn about the psychosocial events involved.
3. Use Bowlby's attachment theory to discuss the impact of grief in this situation.
4. Submit a brief proposal (3–5 pages) for your topic.

Learn about the social work role in helping individuals and families cope with grief and loss by completing the following: Find two or more articles pertaining to your chosen topic in top-tier social work or grief-and-loss scholarly journals. Summarize key features of the articles in one page. (This can be formatted like an annotated bibliography: title of article, source, brief summary of content.) After you have read the textbook and a journal article, interview a social worker (BSW or MSW) who works with clients on issues of grief and loss to learn about the social worker's role, with special emphasis on the clinical insights in helping clients and families cope. This conversation will inform your presentation/discussion of your findings, and your field notes from this conversation will then become part of your paper and your presentation. (On the paper's cover page, please provide the social worker's name and agency.) Examine the social work role in terms of Bowlby's theory, systems theory, or developmental stage theories. This part of your paper should be about four pages.

PRESENTATION OF FIELD NOTES

You will summarize your conversation with the agency social worker who has expertise in the topic under consideration. Feel free to invite your interviewee to attend. (You will also have summarized your discussion in your major paper.)

12

Grief Therapy

Sara Sanders

Conduct two interviews with individuals who have grieved a death and a nondeath-related loss. Identify their experiences with grief, treatments that were utilized, barriers to their grief, things that facilitated their grief, and where they are now as they reflect on the loss. Then, utilizing the various theories of grief, analyze their grief experience in terms of health versus complicated grief issues. Finally, provide a recommendation from a clinical perspective on the types of treatment you feel they should have received and if you feel treatment is necessary now.

13

Topical Seminar in Social Work

End-of-Life Care

Sherri Weisenfluh

FAMILY DISCUSSION AND ANALYSIS

Interview your family members about their views on the choices they would want to make at the end of their lives (e.g., Would you want to be kept alive if a doctor said there was no chance you would regain consciousness?). Using your state's advance directive as a guide, make your own decisions and fill out your own documents. Write a brief paper (3–4 pages) on this experience.

CULTURAL DIFFERENCES IN END-OF-LIFE CARE

Select two different ethnic cultures and do an analysis of how the two groups might differ with respect to issues of health, illness, death, and loss. Detail possible attitudes and beliefs and discuss how you would intervene and help the family as their mother nears death. Give a ten-minute class presentation.

FINAL PROJECT

Pick an ethical issue in end-of-life care. Research the issues, and discuss any relevant laws or regulations surrounding the ethical issue. What spiritual or cultural considerations need to be examined? What values and beliefs do you hold that lead you to take a specific position? (e.g., Should physician-assisted suicide be legal in all states? How should we decide what care to provide if an individual did not make his or her wishes known?)

Part Five

BSW Course Syllabi and Modules

14

Death, Dying, and Bereavement

Jerry Jo Manfred-Gilham

COURSE OBJECTIVES

In this course, the student will:

- Explore human experiences of loss, separation, and death throughout the life course
- Understand the theoretical underpinnings for explaining loss and separation
- Identify the various models of grief
- Examine cultural, ethical, social, emotional, and spiritual issues associated with loss and death
- Understand the process of coping and readjustment
- Learn techniques for assisting individuals and families as they experience loss and death

COURSE DESCRIPTION

This course focuses on the human experiences of loss and death. Skills for personal coping and for professional work assisting others in dealing with loss are presented. Topics covered include death and children; death and the elderly; ethical issues of death and dying; caregiving of the dying; and financial, economic, and legal issues associated with death and dying.

TEXTS

Leming, M. R., & Dickinson, G. E. (2002). *Understanding dying, death, and bereavement* (5th ed.). Fort Worth, TX: Harcourt College.

Sprang, G., & McNeil, J. (1995). *The many faces of bereavement: The nature and treatment of natural, traumatic, and stigmatized grief.* New York: Brunner/Mazel.

RECOMMENDED READING

Parry, J. K., & Ryan, A. S. (Eds.). (1995). *A cross-cultural look at death, dying and religion.* Chicago: Nelson-Hall.

EVALUATION

Journal and Paper	50 points
Papers (2)	50 points each
Midterm	50 points
Final	50 points

ACTIVITIES AND ASSIGNMENTS

1. The purpose of this activity is for you to become aware of everyday situations and feelings regarding loss and death. Keep a record of your daily thoughts regarding loss and death. Document the context for your thoughts and discuss your reflection on the experience. Then write a reflection paper on the journal entries, and discuss how your ideas and beliefs about loss and death have changed over the course of the term.
2. Explore a significant experience related to loss or death and its impact. You should describe the loss, your response, your coping methods, and the response of significant others; identify cultural and spiritual factors that affected your response; and explain your current feelings about the loss.
3. Conduct a field activity related to the course content, and complete a paper regarding the meaning of the activity and your reaction to it. Be sure to address how this experience affected you personally and professionally. You may

    - Visit a nursing home and document your perceptions
    - Interview a terminally ill individual or the family member of a terminally ill patient regarding his or her feelings and thoughts
    - Visit a funeral home and interview a funeral director
    - Attend a grief support group meeting and document your perceptions
    - Accompany a home health or hospice worker on a home visit to an elderly or terminally ill patient
    - Interview a recently divorced individual and an individual who has been divorced for an extended period and compare and contrast their responses
    - Interview an individual who has survived a traumatic event or natural disaster and document his or her response to that event and your perceptions of his or her current coping

Other ideas will be considered but must be approved by the instructor. All these activities should be undertaken with utmost respect for the feelings and confidentiality of others.

COURSE OUTLINE

Session 1	Overview of the course and review of course outline Life course development Theoretical underpinning for examining loss and separation Attitudes regarding death Reading: Leming & Dickinson, chapters 1–3 Activity: Explore euphemisms Exercise: Free association
Session 2	Types of loss—divorce, death, and other separations Reactions to loss—emotional, behavioral, social, and cognitive Models of grief Reading: Sprang & McNeil, pp. 3–11 Activity: Exercise regarding losses
Session 3	Premature or traumatized death Post-traumatic stress disorder Reading: Sprang & McNeil, section 2
Session 4	Stigmatized death Reading: Sprang & McNeil, section 3; Leming & Dickinson, chapter 9 Activity: Film
Session 5	Spirituality and grief Hope and healing Physicians and spirituality Reading: Leming & Dickinson, chapter 4 First examination
Session 6	The dying patient Reading: Leming & Dickinson, chapters 5–6 Activity: Film
Session 7	Health-care issues Reading: Leming & Dickinson, chapter 7 Activity: Speaker
Session 8	Children and death Death of a child Reading: Sprang & McNeil, pp. 26–52; Leming & Dickinson, chapters 3 and 14

Session 9	The elderly and dying Reading: Sprang & McNeil, pp. 12–25 Second examination Activity: Film
Session 10	Bereavement and coping Support systems Self-help groups Reading: Leming & Dickinson, chapter 13 Activity: Film
Session 11	Ethical and moral issues Euthanasia and assisted suicide Reading: Leming & Dickinson, chapter 8 Activity: Debate
Session 12	Ceremony and ritual Funeral arrangements Reading: Leming & Dickinson, chapter 10 Activity: Speaker
Session 13	Culture and death Reading: Leming & Dickinson, chapter 10; Parry & Ryan (all chapters)
Session 14	Legal issues-advance directives, DNR, insurance Reading: Leming & Dickinson, chapter 12
Session 15	Economic issues Reading: Leming & Dickinson, chapter 11; Sprang & McNeil, pp. 12–25

15

Death, Dying, and Bereavement

Lucinda Lee Roff

COURSE DESCRIPTION

This course introduces students to issues and problems presented by death, dying, and grief. Designed for social work majors and others in the helping professions, it examines attitudes and responses to death, the perspectives of dying children and adults, euthanasia, abortion, suicide, capital punishment, funeral behavior, and the dynamics of grief. Students are encouraged to examine and challenge their own values and attitudes and to consider the implications of course content for professional behavior.

OBJECTIVES

Upon successful completion of this course, students should be able to:

- Discuss articulately their own attitudes and feelings about death-related issues
- Discuss how attitudes and experiences with death are influenced by gender, race, ethnicity, culture, class, sexual orientation, mental or physical ability, religion, national origin, and other factors
- Discuss legal, medical, and social definitions of death
- Discuss how dying individuals perceive themselves and the reactions of others around them
- Discuss the processes of normal and dysfunctional grief
- Discuss social work values and ethics in death-related situations
- Discuss social work interventions with dying and bereaved persons
- Discuss suicide, war, abortion, medical technology, euthanasia, violent death, and capital punishment in the context of social and economic justice

TEXT

Kastenbaum, R. J. (2004). *Death, society, and human experience.* Boston: Allyn and Bacon.

REQUIREMENTS AND GRADING

Course requirement	Maximum possible points
Class participation	10
Five short papers (20 each)	100
Quiz 1	45
Quiz 2	45
Final examination	100
Total	300

COURSE OUTLINE

Session 1 Meaning of death (Kastenbaum, chapters 2 and 3)
Paper 1 due

Why do people fear death? What about death do they fear?
How do people accept or deny death?
Do we feel differently about death of the elderly and the death of the young?
What do euphemisms and jokes tell us about our feelings about death?
How do we know when someone is dead? Are people ever buried alive?
Is death an event or a state?
What conditions resemble death, and what conditions does death resemble?
Are there beings that resemble death, personifications of death?
How does death create political and social change?
What are religious aspects of death?

Session 2 Death system (Kastenbaum, chapter 4)
What are definitions of death?
What would it be like if death didn't exist?
What are the components of the death system in U.S. society?
What does each component do?
What has changed the death system in the United States in the last century or so?
What are some of the basics of the demography of death?
What are some social and economic justice issues regarding death?

How are death systems different in non-U.S. cultures?
How is body disposal handled in countries with small land masses?
Are people able to deal financially with a sudden death?

Session 3 Dying process (Kastenbaum, chapter 5)
Paper 2 due

When does dying begin?
How do you tell the bad news?
What are different dying trajectories?
How do people experience the dying process?
What do people do differently when they have a terminal diagnosis?
Do we die in stages?
Do people know they will die soon? What sensations do they have?
Is there such a thing as a peaceful death?

Session 4 Hospice and terminal care (Kastenbaum, chapter 6)
Quiz 1

What's the history of the hospice movement?
What are hospice standards of care?
What does hospice mean by a peaceful death, and how does it attempt to achieve it?
What is done to relieve pain?
What are experiences of hospice patients, staff, and volunteers?

Session 5 End-of-life issues and decisions (Kastenbaum, chapter 7)
Paper 3 due

How can we be sure advance directives are followed?
How do social work values and ethics inform end-of-life decisions?
What is the legal status of various end-of-life documents?
How do race, ethnicity, and culture affect opinions about end-of-life issues?

Session 6 Suicide (Kastenbaum, chapter 8)
Are the people left behind after a suicide survivors or victims?
What can be done to prevent suicide?
What are the statistical facts about suicide in the United States?
What are the reasons why people commit suicide?
What is the role of religion and culture in beliefs about suicide?

Session 7 Violent death (Kastenbaum, chapters 9 and 1)
Paper 4 due

How do mass deaths affect our feelings?
What are the facts about murder in the United States?
Discuss terrorism as an instrument of political and social control.
Under what circumstances do family members kill one another?
What can be done to reduce the murder rate in the United States?
What are the facts about accidental death in the United States?
How does the military train people to kill in wartime?
What is the experience of soldiers in wartime and after their return home?
What is the impact of 9/11 and similar events?

Session 8 Assisted death (Kastenbaum, chapter 10)
Is assisted suicide ethical? Under what circumstances?
What are the pros and cons of assisted death (euthanasia)?
How do social work values inform decisions about assisted suicide?
What is the history of assisted suicide in the United States?
What are the provisions of the assisted suicide law in the Netherlands?
What are the provisions of the assisted suicide law in Oregon?

Session 9 Death and children (Kastenbaum, chapter 11)
Quiz 2
How does one explain death to a child?
How can we help children deal with funerals and the grieving process?
How do children conceptualize death at different ages?
What interventions are used with children who are dying?
How are children affected by images of war, violence, and terrorism?
How do parents deal with a child's death?
How does losing a parent affect young children?

Session 10 Bereavement, grief, and mourning (Kastenbaum, chapter 12)
How do we help others cope with death?
Do people die of a broken heart?
How is bereavement handled in different cultures?
How do you prepare for a loved one's death?
Is seeing the body important?

Session 11 The funeral process (Kastenbaum, chapter 13)
What is the technical procedure for preparing a body?
What are cultural differences in funeral ceremonies and grieving?
Why is only the top part of the body seen in caskets?
How do post-funeral customs differ regionally?

Can we plan our own funerals?
What affects the costs of funerals?
What is embalming all about?
What happens during cremation?
How are funerals handled when the body is disfigured?

SHORT PAPERS

Each paper should be 350–500 words.

Paper 1: Discuss the experiences in your past that have most significantly influenced your current attitudes and feelings about death. Explain how these experiences have had an important influence. Consider your entire life history (from early childhood to present) as you prepare to answer this question.

Paper 2: Explain how your life would change if you learned you had a life-threatening illness from which your were likely to die within a year.

Paper 3: Have you made or will you make an advance directive? Describe your thought processes in thinking about this question, and explain your decision. Give attention to any barriers or resistance you may be encountering in thinking about making an advance directive.

Paper 4: Under what circumstances, if any, is it good or desirable for our government to execute one of its citizens?

Paper 5: Describe a public funeral process (e.g., a wake, funeral/memorial service, burial/cremation, activities following disposal of remains) in which you have participated. Discuss your impressions and reactions. To what extent did this process help you accept and adjust to the loss of the deceased? Or, imagine you will die within the next year. Explain in detail the funeral process (including wake, funeral/memorial service, burial/cremation, and activities following disposal of your remains) that you would like to have conducted in your memory. Explain the reasons for your wishes.

16

Death and Dying

Sheila Gillespie Roth

COURSE DESCRIPTION

This course provides a consideration of the current state of clinical and social science knowledge of the death-and-dying experience of individuals and families. Students consider the individual and family dynamics of death and grief; the origin of American health-care systems centered around death; the phenomenon of grief and bereavement; and ethical issues of death, euthanasia, and suicide.

TEXT

Albom, M. (1997). *Tuesdays with Morrie*. New York: Bantam Doubleday Dell.

COURSE OBJECTIVES

The student will

- Develop an understanding of how our thoughts and feelings about death develop from childhood
- Increase his or her knowledge of potential death issues such as living with AIDS, physician-assisted death, suicide, homicide, and terrorism
- Develop an understanding of the differences in the ways people respond to the challenges of grieving and dying
- Acquire knowledge of skills that are useful in supporting the grieving person
- Increase his or her understanding of the cross-cultural aspects of death and dying
- Develop an awareness of his or her own feelings about death issues

ASSIGNMENTS AND ACTIVITIES

Each student will read the book *Tuesdays with Morrie.* You will think critically about and analyze the key relationships that evolve and the messages that emerge about life, dying, and death. The paper should be written with the above considerations in mind. This paper must be typed and double spaced. Please do not exceed five pages.

Memory box: Each student will make a box of remembrance for someone or some part of his or her life in which there has been a loss. The box can be a decorated shoebox or cigar box. It can also be an envelope. The idea is for the student to place items in the box that evoke memories of that loss. The box will be a stimulus for classroom discussion of feelings, memories, and healing. Students need not share the memory box with the class but may if the instructor and student believe that it is appropriate.

Drawing in grief: This is a role-play exercise in which students draw (in the mind-set of a child) what grief looks like. The student playing the social worker will talk with the child about the feelings brought up by the drawing.

Attitudes on aging: Students will discuss their thoughts and beliefs about aging. Journal writing will be discussed as a way for individuals to reflect on aging, growth, love, and lessons learned from life experiences.

Midterm paper: Each student will be required to explore a belief system other than his or her own by writing a paper of at least eight to ten pages discussing death as it is viewed from that belief system. This paper must be typed (double spaced) and should include proper citations and a reference list. Each student will present his or her paper to the class.

Final paper: This semester-long reflection paper will be an analytical reflection of self-growth. This semester we will be exploring important issues in relation to dying, death, and bereavement. Each student will keep a journal on his or her experiences during the course (i.e., lectures, guest speakers, field trips). The information from your journal should be supplemented in the paper with information from books and journals. Questions to ask yourself during the semester are: (1) What new knowledge or valuable information did I learn from the lectures, speakers, and field trips? (2) What death-related issues are specific to children, adolescents, adults, or the elderly? (3) Did I learn new information about funerals, rituals, and preparing for death? (4) What did I learn about my own thoughts in relation to dying and death? (5) What impact does death have on culture or vice versa? (6) Have your relationships with others changed as a result of this knowledge? (7) What coping skills do I have for times of bereavement? (8) How can I help others who are in mourning? This paper should be reflective and factual. It should be approximately ten pages in length.

COURSE OUTLINE

Session 1 What is loss?
What is death?
Grief and bereavement defined
Reading: Begin *Tuesdays with Morrie*

Session 2 Attitudes about loss and dying
Self-inventory exercise: Death Anxiety Scale in Aiken
Discussion: I am afraid of . . .

Session 3 Bereavement and mourning
Reading: "Grieving Process" and "Grief and Depression Are Intimate Strangers" in Leming & Dickinson
Help in the process
Reading: "Grief Tips" in Leming & Dickinson

Session 4 Stages of death and dying (Kübler-Ross)
Tuesdays with Morrie papers due

Session 5 Film: *Death and Dying: The Physician's Perspective*

Session 6 Guest speaker: Hospice employee

Session 7 Types of death
Accidental/sudden death, terrorism, a long-term illness
Differences in the mourning process related to type of death.

Session 8 Coping and caring
Sharing the story as healing
Role play
Class exercise: Loss history
Active listening
Nonverbal supports

Session 9 Suicide
The impact of suicide
Suicide intervention

Session 10 Paper presentation
Midterm paper due

Session 11 Gender differences and grieving
Cultural differences and death

Session 12 Guest speaker: Local SIDS Alliance
Complicated mourning

Reading: "The Increasing Prevalence of Complicated Mourning: The Onslaught Is Just the Beginning" and "Disenfranchised Grief" in Leming & Dickinson
Disenfranchised grief

Session 13 Grieving throughout the life cycle
Childhood and death: Infant to school age
Reading: "Communication among Children, Parents and Funeral Directors" and "Children, Death, and Fairy Tales" in Leming & Dickinson
Exercise: Drawing in grief

Session 14 Adolescence and young adulthood
Exercise: Memory box

Session 15 Adulthood and the elder years
Journal writing as a coping tool
Exercise: Attitudes on aging

Session 16 Presentation of memory boxes
Discussion

Session 17 Legal issues
Living wills
Durable power of attorney in health care

Session 18 Guest speaker: Funeral director

Session 19 Film: *Juveniles and the Death Penalty*

Session 20 Coroner's office tour/speaker

Session 21 Discussion and review of coroner's office tour/speaker and related issues

Session 22 Guest speaker (Muslim perspective)

Session 23 Guest speaker (Buddhist perspective)

Session 24 Guest speaker (Jewish perspective)

Session 25 Final paper presentations

BIBLIOGRAPHY

Aiken, L. (1994). *Dying, death and bereavement* (3rd ed.). Boston: Allyn and Bacon.

Aldwin, Carolyn. (1994). *Stress, coping, and development*. New York: Guilford Press.

Astor, R., Behre, W., Wallace, J., & Fravil, K. (1998). School social workers and school violence: Personal safety, training, and violence programs. *Social Work, 43*(6), 223–232.

Barker, R. L. (1991). *The social work dictionary*. Silver Springs, MD: NASW Press.

Blumenthal, S., & Kupfer, D. (1990). *Suicide over the life cycle: Risk factors, assessment, and treatment of suicidal patients.* Washington, DC: American Psychiatric Press.

Csikai, E., & Chaitin, E. (2006). *Ethics in end-of-life decisions in social work practice.* Chicago: Lyceum Books.

Faul, A., & Hudson, W. (1997). The index of drug involvement: A partial validation. *Social Work, 42*(6), 565–572.

Hatfield, A. (1990). *Family education in mental illness.* New York: Guilford Press.

Hendricks, J. (1991). *Crisis intervention in criminal justice/social service.* Springfield, IL: C. C. Thomas.

Lefley, H., & Pedersen, P. (1992). *Cross-cultural training for mental health professionals.* Springfield, IL: C. C. Thomas.

Leming, M. R., & Dickinson, G. E. (1999). *Understanding dying, death, and bereavement.* Guilford, CT: Dushkin.

Lewis, J., Hayes, B., & Bradley, L. (1992). *Counseling women over the lifespan.* Denver, CO: Love Publishing.

Mannino, J. D. (1997). *Grieving days, healing days.* Boston: Allyn and Bacon.

Nicholas, M. P. (1995). *The lost art of listening.* New York: Guilford Press.

Parry, J., & Ryan, A. (1995). *A cross-cultural look at death, dying, and religion.* Chicago: Nelson-Hall.

Pfeiffer, C. (1989). *Suicide among youth: Perspectives on risk and prevention.* Washington, DC: American Psychiatric Press.

Webb, N. B. (1996). *Social work practice with children.* New York: Guilford Press.

Wehrly, B. (1995). *Pathways to multicultural counseling competence.* Pacific Grove, CA: Brooks Cole.

17

Social Work with the Dying and Their Families

Five Curriculum Modules for Educating the Generalist Practitioner

Cheryl Brandsen and Mary Carlsen

End-of-life care has become a subject of increasing importance to social workers. It is not uncommon for social workers in a variety of practice settings to work with individuals who are facing life-threatening conditions, individuals who are dying, and individuals who are grieving. These modules will assist undergraduate social work faculty in their instruction of beginning generalist practitioners. This preparation is crucial to undergraduate education. The modules presented here are introductory, broad, and flexible; they have sufficient depth and specificity to measurably improve students' knowledge and skills in end-of-life care.

The effort to write these curriculum modules was aided by many sources noted in the bibliography. Additionally, we are grateful for the support of the Robert Wood Johnson Foundation, which funded state partnerships in Michigan and Minnesota to improve end-of-life care. The modules were developed in response to statewide surveys and interviews that addressed practitioners' needs for education related to end-of-life care.

The following assumptions are foundational to the use of these curriculum modules:

- Nonmedical strengths-based principles of practice are central to all modules.
- These stand-alone modules can be integrated into a variety of courses in BSW programs. While it seems most logical that they would be used in practice courses, these modules have also been used in policy, HBSE, and ethics courses. The timing and placement of the modules are left up to the discretion of individual instructors or curriculum committees.

- The curriculum is designed to provide a basic overview to educate beginning generalist practitioners (i.e., the young and/or new practitioner with little or no practice wisdom or experience); it is not intended to be used as specialist preparation.
- The general focus is on preparing students to work with issues related to dying, death, and bereavement in any practice setting (i.e., elementary school children, elderly prisoners, foster children, individuals with mental health problems and developmental disabilities), not solely those settings related to health care.
- Many exercises are provided, but these are not exhaustive. Other types of experiential exercises are available from local hospices and the health and social work literature.
- The modules are flexibly designed, with no time limits. Instructors can tailor each module to classes lasting one to two hours, depending on instructor expertise and the level of student ability and experience.

The following five topics are addressed here:

- Macro issues in end of life
- Personal comfort in working with the dying
- The dying experience
- Loss, grief, and bereavement
- The intersection of ethics, practice, and policy in end-of-life care

Each module is structured in the following way: pre-class assignment, learning objectives, lecture outline, instructional resources, bibliography, webliography, and evaluation.

Some general suggestions for overall implementation of these modules:

Discuss with students the reasons for the inclusion of this content in the social work curriculum:

- All social workers will face these issues in practice.
- Little preparation is available to students in baccalaureate social work programs in the United States.
- Social workers have special expertise to share with other professionals and with those who are dying and their family members.
- High-quality compassionate care of the dying and their loved ones should be a goal of social work education and practice.

For evaluation, consider having students rate themselves on the objectives at the beginning of the class and again once the course has ended.

While each module includes possible bibliographic supplements, a more complete bibliography is provided at the end.

Module 1: Macro Issues in End-of-Life Care

PRE-CLASS ASSIGNMENT

Consult the module bibliography and instructional resources for possible pre-class reading and/or assignments.

LEARNING OBJECTIVES

Upon completion of this module, students will:

- Understand definitions of end of life
- Understand the demographics, trends, and major social issues related to death and dying
- Understand the different services available people at the end of their lives
- Understand the relationship of end-of-life issues to various social work practice settings
- Understand several social policy issues in death and dying

LECTURE OUTLINE

1. History of end of life
   a. Dying looks much different in 2005 than it did one hundred years ago (Lynn et al., 2000).
   b. Introduction of hospice care in the United States.
2. Defining the period of time known as "end of life"
   a. This definition has expanded in recent years to include approximately the last two years before death.
   b. The Medicare Hospice Benefit restricts the definition of "end of life" to the last six months of life
   c. When would you consider yourself to be dying? When you had two years to live? One year to live? Six months? One day?
   d. Would you ever want to be labeled as dying while you were still living?
3. Demographics and trends (National Center, 2002)
   a. In 1999, 2,391,399 people died in the United States
   b. Leading causes of death in the United States
   c. Statewide demographics
   d. Death demographics by race

4. Contemporary end-of-life issues
   a. Treatment of pain and suffering
   b. Advance care planning
   c. Physician-assisted suicide / euthanasia
   d. Access to services for the dying / who pays for care at the end of life?
   e. Societal fears of discussing death
   f. Cultural differences in beliefs about death and dying
   g. End of life in the courts
5. End-of-life care sites and problems in dying

   Sites of death: Acute care, home care with and without hospice, nursing homes
6. Additional sources of help for the dying and their families
   a. Mutual aid / informal services
   b. Community-based services
7. Social work and end-of-life care
   a. All social workers need to have an awareness of issues related to death and grief. It is a requirement that we have self-awareness in practice; this is particularly important where dying and grieving are concerned.
   b. All practice settings have potential for practice with death or grief; an interdisciplinary approach to care is important.
   c. Social workers have special expertise in assessing strengths; empowering individuals, families, and communities; intervening to improve social functioning; and working for policy changes to improve people's lives. This strengths approach is very different from a deficits, pathology, or medical model of pathology, diagnosis, and treatment.
   d. It is the obligation of social workers to see that clients who are dying, grieving, or bereaved, and their families, get connected to appropriate resources to assist them. If those resources do not exist, or clients do not have the means to access them, it is the role of the social worker to address that gap.
   e. Social workers are expected to go into the community and provide assistance to clients who are dying or grieving. However, social workers are poorly trained by educational institutions to perform this role.
   f. There is limited data regarding the value of social work in end-of-life care. Social workers have a responsibility to complete empirical studies to demonstrate their value to persons facing death, to their families, and to the organizations providing services.

INSTRUCTIONAL RESOURCES

Small Group Activities

Assign students in small groups a nonmedical practice setting (e.g., child protection, school, foster care, camp, adoption agency, senior services, criminal justice/corrections, emergency services, basic needs agencies). Ask each group to discuss these questions: In what ways might end-of-life issues arise for social work clients in this setting? Consider possible scenarios for an individual, a group, a family, the organization, and/or the community it serves. Students should write down all possibilities and be prepared to share at least two situations with the class.

In small groups, have students discuss this scenario and report back to the larger group: "You are considered an expert in the field of end-of-life care. You have been invited to visit (city/state), which has a population of ________, to give advice to the ministry of health on what services are required for people at the end of life." Provide students with various fact sheets related to end-of-life care with information such as the roles of social workers in end-of-life settings, statewide resource kits on end-of-life care, and myths and facts about end-of-life care. The student report to the larger group should address services and gaps in service delivery.

Additional Assignment Options

1. Interview social workers in nonmedical practice settings about end-of-life care.
2. Complete a literature search on a specific macro issue in end of life.
3. Observe an ethics committee deliberation at a local agency.
4. Research issues in end-of-life care for a specific population at risk.

Discussion Questions

1. What are some of the hopeful trends in end of life in the United States? (Consider legal right to advance care planning, longer life span, hospice care, etc.)
2. Where might some gaps in services exist for people who are dying or grieving? (Consider rural or poor communities.)
3. What are the most controversial issues in death and dying? Why do you think they are controversial?
4. Why is it important for social workers to have knowledge and skill in end-of-life care?

Handouts

Norlander, L., & Baines, B. K. (2003). The five guiding principles for end of life care: Minnesota's framework. *Home Health Care Management & Practice, 15*(2), 110–115.

Problems in end-of-life care. (2000, May). Information Sheet for the Minnesota Commission on End-of-Life Care.

BIBLIOGRAPHY

Amar, D. F. (1994). The role of the hospice social worker in the nursing home setting. *American Journal of Hospice and Palliative Care, 11*(3), 18–22.

Baker, M. E. (2000). Knowledge and attitudes of health care social workers regarding advance directives. *Social Work in Health Care, 32,* 61–74.

Becker, J. E. (2004). Oncology social workers' attitudes toward hospice care and referral behavior. *Health and Social Work, 29,* 36–45.

Bern-Klug, M., Ekerdt, D. J., & Wilkinson, D. S. (1999). What families know about funeral-related costs: Implications for social work practice. *Health and Social Work, 24*(2), 128–137.

Bern-Klug, M., Gessert, C., & Forbes, S. (2001). The need to revise assumptions about the end of life: Implications for social work practice. *Health and Social Work, 26*(1), 38–48.

Botsford, A. L. (2000). Integrating end-of-life care into services for people with an intellectual disability. *Social Work in Health Care, 31*(1), 35–48.

Brandsen, C. K. (2005). Social work and end-of-life care: Reviewing the past and moving forward. *Journal of Social Work in End-of-Life and Palliative Care, 1*(2), 45–70.

Care at the End of Life. (2000). *Best practice series: Innovative practice in social work.* Philadelphia: Society for Social Work Leadership in Health Care.

Casarett, D. J., Karlawish, J. H. T., & Byock, I. (2002). Advocacy and activism: Missing pieces in the quest to improve end-of-life care. *Journal of Palliative Medicine, 5,* 3–12.

Christ, G., & Blacker, S. (2005). Setting an agenda for social work in end-of-life care: An overview of leadership and organizational initiatives. *Journal of Social Work in End-of-Life and Palliative Care, 1*(1), 9–17.

Chichin, E. R., Ferster, L., & Gordon, N. (1994). Planning for the end of life with the home care client. *Journal of Gerontological Social Work, 22*(1/2), 147–159.

Csikai, E. L. (2004). Social workers' participation in the resolution of ethical dilemmas in hospice care. *Health and Social Work, 29,* 67–76.

Csikai, E. L., & Bass, K. (2000). Health care social workers' views of ethical issues, practice, and policy in end-of-life care. *Social Work in Health Care, 32*(2), 1–22.

Csikai, E. L., & Manetta, A. A. (2002). Preventing unnecessary deaths among older adults: A call to action for social workers. *Journal of Gerontological Social Work, 38,* 85–97.

Dungan, S. S., Jaquay, T. R., Rezink, K. A., & Sands, E. A. (1995). Pediatric critical care social work: Clinical practice with parents of critically ill children. *Social Work in Health Care, 21*(1), 69–80.

Egan, M., & Kadushin, G. (1999). The social worker in the emerging field of home care: Professional activities and ethical concerns. *Health and Social Work, 24*(1), 43–55.

Galambos, C. M. (1998). Preserving end-of-life autonomy: The Patient Self-Determination Act and the Uniform Health Care Decisions Act. *Health and Social Work, 23*(4), 275–281.

Gunter-Hunt, G., Mahoney, J. E., & Sieger, C. E. (2002). A comparison of state advance directive documents. *The Gerontologist, 42,* 51–60.

Gwyther, L. P., Altilio, T., Blacker, S., Christ, G., Csikai, E. L., Hooyman, N., et al. (2005). Social work competencies in palliative and end-of-life care. *Journal of Social Work in End-of-Life and Palliative Care, 1,* 87–120.

Kovacs, P. J., & Bronstein, L. R. (1999). Preparation for oncology settings: What hospice social workers say they need. *Health and Social Work, 24*(1), 57–64.

Luptak, M. (2004). Social work and end-of-life care for older people: A historical perspective. *Health and Social Work, 29,* 7–15.

Mezey, M., Mitty, E., Rappaport, M., & Ramsey, G. (1997). Implementation of the Patient Self-Determination Act (PSDA) in nursing homes in New York City. *Journal of the American Geriatrics Society, 45*(1), 43–49.

National Association of Social Workers. (2000). *Social work speaks: NASW policy statements.* Washington, DC: NASW Press.

Neuman, K., & Wade, L. (1999). Advance directives: The experience of health care professionals across the continuum of care. *Social Work in Health Care, 28*(3), 39–54.

Quinn, A. (1998). Learning from palliative care: Concepts to underpin the transfer of knowledge from specialist palliative care to mainstream social work settings. *Social Work Education, 17*(1), 9–20.

Reese, D. J., Ahern, R. E., Nair, S., O'Faire, J. D., & Warren, C. (1999). Hospice access and use by African Americans: Addressing cultural and institutional barriers through participatory action research. *Social Work, 44*(6), 549–559.

Reese, D. J., & Raymer, M. (2004). Relationships between social work involvement and hospice outcomes: Results of the national hospice social work survey. *Social Work, 49,* 415–422.

Remsen, M. F. (1993). The role of the nursing home social worker in terminal care. *Journal of Gerontological Social Work, 19*(3/4), 193–205.

Rice, J. R., Hicks, P. B., & Wiehe, V. (2000). Life care planning: A role for social workers. *Social Work in Health Care, 31*(1), 85–94.

Roff, S. (2001). Analyzing end-of-life care legislation: A social work perspective. *Social Work in Health Care, 33,* 51–68.

Sheldon, F. M. (2000). Dimensions of the role of the social worker in palliative care. *Palliative Medicine, 14*(6), 491–498.

Stein, G. L. (2004). Improving our care at life's end: Making a difference. *Health and Social Work, 29,* 77–79.

Stoesen, L. (2002). Role in end-of-life care examined. *NASW News, 47*(5), 4.

Taylor-Brown, S., Teeter, J. A., & Blackburn, E. (1998). Parental loss due to HIV: Caring for children as a community issue—the Rochester, New York experience. *Child Welfare, 77*(2), 137–160.

Werth, J. L. (2002). Legal and ethical considerations for mental health professionals related to end-of-life care and decision making. *American Behavioral Scientist, 46,* 373–383.

Werth, J. L., & Blevins, D. (2002). Public policy and end-of-life care. *American Behavioral Scientist, 46,* 401–417.

Werth, J. L., Blevins, D., Toussaint, K. L., & Durham, M. R. (2002). The influence of cultural diversity on end-of-life care and decisions. *American Behavioral Scientist, 46,* 204–219.

Wesley, C. A. (1996). Social work and end-of-life decisions: Self-determination and the common good. *Health and Social Work, 21*(2), 115–121.

WEBLIOGRAPHY

Centers for Disease Control: http://www.cdc.gov/nchs/data/dvs/nvsr53_17tableE2002.pdf

Brown University Center for Gerontology and Health Care Research: http://www.chcr.brown.edu

Last Acts Organization: http://www.lastacts.org

Minnesota Partnership: http://www.minnesotapartnership.org/guidprin.htm

National Center for Health Statistics: http://www.cdc.gov

Robert Wood Johnson Foundation: http://www.rwjf.org

World Federation of Right to Die Societies: http://www.worldrtd.net

EVALUATION

1. Self-evaluation (have students rank themselves on module learning objectives; see evaluation form)
2. Quiz on lecture material
3. Pre/post-test of students' knowledge

Module 2: Personal Comfort in Working with the Dying

PRE-CLASS ASSIGNMENT

Consult module bibliography and instructional resources for possible pre-class readings and/or assignments

LEARNING OBJECTIVES

The goal of this module is for students:

- To explore their own values about death and dying to assess readiness to begin practice
- To recognize the richness and value in the experiences of loss and dying
- To gain personal and professional confidence regarding end-of-life practice
- To be able to describe two strategies for self-care

LECTURE OUTLINE

1. Introduction

   The instructor might share a personal story about practice with the dying that illustrates his or her own fears and humanity or a boundary issue (e.g., receiving a gift) rather than "showing off" the best practice; the instructor could also share a bit of his or her own loss history so students feel they have permission to share their own personal stories; the instructor might read a social work narrative before class.
2. Personal feelings and values about death and dying
   a. Dying is a rich stage in the life cycle, one of growth and reflection.
   b. Social workers must know their own loss history and recognize unresolved issues.
   c. Social workers should model advance care planning.
3. Types of losses (related to dying, death, secondary losses, etc.)
4. Importance of the social worker's confidence in identifying, assessing, and intervening where death and grief issues occur, regardless of practice setting
   a. Naming potential or actual loss or grief
   b. Assessment of whether the loss issues are barriers to full functioning in the setting

   c. Use of self-awareness, nonjudgmental attitude, and strengths assessment of client's biopsychosocial-spiritual whole to ensure we don't miss client needs due to our own blind spots
   d. Practice overview
   e. Importance of self-knowledge
   f. Cultural differences related to end-of-life care and grieving (be sure to illustrate relevant local cultural differences)

5. Importance and difficulty of self-care, regardless of how experienced one is
   a. Physical and emotional care of oneself
   b. Processing feelings/experience with someone while respecting confidentiality
   c. Institutional assistance for professional work
   d. Formation of network of support with social workers doing similar work
   e. Importance of continuing education in this area
7. Signs of burnout (see Sheafor, Horseji, & Horseji, pp. 213–216)

INSTRUCTIONAL RESOURCES

Exercises

1. Self-awareness exercise: "I Am Afraid of Dying" (Mannino, p. 16)
2. Personal object exercise (bring in an object related to the person who dies and talk about it)
3. Death anxiety scale exercise (Mannino, p. 18, or Leming)
4. Timeline of loss
5. Course intake assessment (Mannino, pp. 220–222)
6. Loss history (Worden)

Discussion Questions

1. What internal or external resources have you used in your life to cope with losses you have experienced? What strengths might you bring to this area of practice?
2. What do you think will be the most difficult part of practice with end of life for you?
3. How might you continue your efforts to increase your personal and professional comfort in end-of-life practice after this class?
4. What strategies for self-care might work best for you, and why? What additional strategies might you share with the group?

Assignments

1. Attempt a draft of an ethical will or an advance directive for yourself (www.fivewishes.org).
2. Interview a social worker who works with the dying. Ask about how he or she copes with the emotional toll of caring for the dying, what he or she has learned from working with the dying, and how he or she cares for him- or herself.
3. Attend the funeral of a person whose cultural background differs from your own (must be approved by instructor).

BIBLIOGRAPHY

Baines, B. (2001). *Putting your values on paper: The ethical will writing guide workbook.* Minneapolis, MN: Josaba.

Becker, J. E. (2004). Oncology social workers' attitudes toward hospice care and referral behavior. *Health and Social Work, 29,* 36–45.

Csikai, E. L. (1999). Euthanasia and assisted suicide: Issues for social work practice. *Journal of Gerontological Social Work, 31*(3/4), 49–63.

Csikai, E. L. (1999). Hospital social worker attitudes toward euthanasia and assisted suicide. *Social Work in Health Care, 30*(1), 57–73.

Csikai, E. L. (1999). The role of values and experience in determining social workers' attitudes toward euthanasia and assisted suicide. *Social Work in Health Care, 30*(1), 75–95.

Csikai, E. L., & Bass, K. (2000). Health care social workers' views of ethical issues, practice, and policy in end-of-life care. *Social Work in Health Care, 32*(2), 1–22.

Davidson, K. W., & Foster, Z. (1995). Social work with dying and bereaved clients: Helping the workers. *Social Work in Health Care, 21*(4), 1–16.

Eftink, S. (n.d.). *Breaking free of fear to lead a better life now: Handbook of twelve death awareness exercises, based on Worden and Proctor.* Unpublished manuscript. Available from seftink@olemiss.edu

Foster, A., & Davidson, K. (1995). Satisfactions and stresses for the social worker. In I. Corless, B. B. Germino, & M. A. Pittman-Lindman (Eds.), *Dying, death, and bereavement: A challenge for living* (pp. 285–300). Boston: Jones and Bartlett.

Kovacs, P. J., & Bronstein, L. R. (1999). Preparation for oncology settings: What hospice social workers say they need. *Health and Social Work, 24*(1), 57–64.

Kramer, B. J. (1998). Preparing social workers for the inevitable: A preliminary investigation of a course on grief, death, and loss. *Journal of Social Work Education, 34,* 211–227.

Leichtentritt, R. D., & Rettig, K. D. (2001). Values underlying end-of-life decisions: A qualitative approach. *Health and Social Work, 26,* 150–159.

Mannino, J. D. (1997). *Grieving days, healing days.* Needham Heights, MA: Allyn and Bacon.

Nakashima, M. (1995). Spiritual growth through hospice social work. *Reflections, 1*(4), 17–27.

Neuman, K. (1998). Not the time: A personal reflection on counseling families on end-of-life decisions. *Reflections.* NASW Press.

Peterson, M. (1992). *At personal risk: Boundary violations in professional-client relationships*. New York: W. W. Norton.
Roberts, C. S., Baile, W. F., & Bassett, J. D. (1999). When the care giver needs care. *Social Work in Health Care, 30*(2), 65–80.
Sheafor, B., Horesji, C., & Horesji, G. (2000). *Techniques and guidelines for social work practice* (5th ed.). Boston: Allyn and Bacon.
Smith, S. H. (1999). "Now that Mom is in the Lord's arms, I just have to live the way she taught me": Reflections on an elderly, African American mother's death. *Journal of Gerontological Social Work, 32*(2), 41–51.
Tobin, D. (1998, December). *Peaceful dying: The step-by-step guide to preserving your dignity, your choice, and your inner peace at the end of life*. Reading, MA: Perseus.
Werner, P., Carmel, S., & Ziedenberg, H. (2004). Nurses' and social workers' attitudes and beliefs about and involvement in life-sustaining treatment decisions. *Health and Social Work, 29,* 27–35.
Worden, J. W. (1991). *Grief counseling and grief therapy* (2nd ed.). New York: Spring.

WEBLIOGRAPHY

Aging with Dignity: http://www.fivewishes.org
Ethical Wills: Preserving Your Legacy of Values: http://www.ethicalwill.com

EVALUATION

1. Self-evaluation (have students rank themselves on module learning objectives; see evaluation form)
2. Quiz on lecture material
3. Faculty to evaluate strengths and weaknesses of this module, with suggestions for improvement

Module 3: The Dying Experience

PRE-CLASS ASSIGNMENT

Consult module bibliography and instructional resources for possible pre-class reading and/or assignments.

LEARNING OBJECTIVES

Upon completion of this module, students will be able to:

- Understand the basic physiological process of dying
- Be able to describe categories in a complete psychosocial assessment of dying individuals and their families.
- Understand a range of psychosocial and case management interventions commonly needed by people at the end of life and their loved ones
- Be able to recognize cultural differences in the dying experience

LECTURE OUTLINE

1. Process of dying
   a. Definitions of death
   b. Physiological process of dying (biological systems); signs of impending death
   c. Dying trajectories (only known for some diseases, e.g., cancer)
2. Overview of strengths and needs of people at end of life and their families
   a. Strengths and needs of the individual who is dying
   b. Strengths and needs of the family/loved ones
   c. Importance of documentation (specifics are dependent upon setting)
3. Strategies for social work intervention in end of life
   a. Description of communication guidelines
   b. Communication with the interdisciplinary team (Reese & Brown, 1997)
   c. Case management / community resource availability
   d. Discussion of cultural differences

INSTRUCTIONAL RESOURCES

Class Activities

1. Have students review a film clip or case study illustrating one or more of the above issues (e.g., Moyers's *On Our Own Terms* at www.pbs.org/onourownterms).
2. Show pictures of dying people or invite in a person who is dying.
3. Discuss an advance care planning case study with prompt questions.
4. Complete an exercise with interdisciplinary team (individual roles).
5. Discuss case studies that focus on assessment of strengths and needs.

Discussion Questions

1. What questions might a social worker ask a dying or grieving person in order to assess client strengths?
2. What questions about the experience of dying do you have? Where and how might you find answers to those questions or help others to find answers, or at least some methods to address the questions?

Assignments

1. Complete your own funeral planning.
2. Visit a funeral home to research methods of serving families.
3. Research end-of-life care or end-of-life decision making with a diverse population.

BIBLIOGRAPHY

Arnold, E. M. (2004). Factors that influence consideration of hastening death among people with life-threatening illnesses. *Health and Social Work, 29,* 17–26.

Bern-Klug, M. (2004). The ambiguous dying syndrome. *Health and Social Work, 29,* 55–65.

Care at the End of Life. (2000). *Best practice series: Innovative practice in social work.* Philadelphia: Society for Social Work Leadership in Health Care.

Christ, G., & Blacker, S. (2005). Setting an agenda for social work in end-of-life care: An overview of leadership and organizational initiatives. *Journal of Social Work in End-of-Life and Palliative Care, 1*(1), 9–17.

Connor, S. R., Egan, K. A., Kwilosz, D. M., Larson, D. G., & Reese, D. J. (2002). Interdisciplinary approaches to assisting with end-of-life care and decision making. *American Behavioral Scientist, 46,* 340–356.

Cowles, L. A., & Lefcowitz, M. J. (1992). Interdisciplinary expectations of the medical social worker in the hospital setting. *Health and Social Work, 17,* 57–65.

Csikai, E. L. (2002). The state of hospice ethics committees and the social work role. *Omega: Journal of Death and Dying, 45,* 261–275.

Csikai, E. L. (2004). Social workers' participation in the resolution of ethical dilemmas in hospice care. *Health and Social Work, 29,* 67–76.

Csikai, E. L., & Bass, K. (2000). Health care social workers' views of ethical issues, practice, and policy in end-of-life care. *Social Work in Health Care, 32*(2), 1–22.

Foster, L. W., & McLellan, L. J. (2002). Translating psychosocial insight into ethical discussions supportive of families in end-of-life decision making. *Social Work in Health Care, 35,* 37–51.

Gray, S. W., Zide, M. R., & Wilker, H. (2000). Using the solution focused brief therapy model with bereavement groups in rural communities: Resiliency at its best. *Hospice Journal, 15,* 13–30.

Gwyther, L. P., Altilio, T., Blacker, S., Christ, G., Csikai, E. L., Hooyman, N., et al. (2005). Social work competencies in palliative and end-of-life care. *Journal of Social Work in End-of-Life and Palliative Care, 1,* 87–120.

Kristjanson, L., Dudgeon, D., Nelson, F., Henteleff, P., & Balneaves, L. (1997). Evaluation of an interdisciplinary training program in palliative care: Addressing the needs of rural and northern communities. *Journal of Palliative Care, 13*(3), 5–12.

Landau, R. (1996). Preparing for sudden death or organ donation: An ethical dilemma in social work. *International Social Work, 39,* 431.

Miller, P. J., Hedlund, S. C., & Murphy, K. A. (1998). Social work assessment at end of life: Practice guidelines for suicide and the terminally ill. *Social Work in Health Care, 26*(4), 23–26.

Miller, P. J., Mesler, M. A., & Eggman, S. T. (2002). Take some time to look inside their hearts: Hospice social workers contemplate physician assisted suicide. *Social Work in Health Care, 35*(3), 53–64.

Mizrahi, T., & Abramson, J. (1985). Sources of strain between physicians and social workers: Implications for social workers in health care settings. *Social Work in Health Care, 10*(3), 33–51.

Pauw, M. (1991). The social worker's role with a fetal demise and stillbirth. *Health and Social Work, 16,* 291–297.

Reese, D. J., & Brown, D. R. (1997). Psychosocial and spiritual care in hospice: Differences between nursing, social work, and clergy. *Hospice Journal, 12*(1), 29–41.

Reese, D. J., & Sontag, M. (2001). Successful interprofessional collaboration on the hospice team. *Health and Social Work, 26,* 167–175.

Taylor-Brown, S., Teeter, J. A., & Blackburn, E. (1998). Parental loss due to HIV: Caring for children as a community issue—the Rochester, New York experience. *Child Welfare, 77*(2), 137–160.

Van Bloch, L. (1996). Breaking the bad news when sudden death occurs. *Social Work in Health Care, 23*(4), 91–97.

Van Loon, R. A. (1999). Desire to die in terminally ill people: A framework for assessment and intervention. *Health and Social Work, 24*(4), 260–268.

Wells, P. J. (1993). Preparing for sudden death: Social work in the emergency room. *Social Work, 38,* 339–342.

Wesley, C., Tunney, K., & Duncan, E. (2004). Educational needs of hospice social workers: Spiritual assessment and interventions with diverse populations. *American Journal of Hospital Palliative Care, 21,* 40–46.

WEBLIOGRAPHY

Aging with Dignity: http://www.agingwithdignity.org
End of Life / Palliative Resource Education Center: http://www.eperc.mcw.edu
Hospice Association of America: http://www.hospice-america.org

EVALUATION

1. Self-evaluation (have students rank themselves on module learning objectives; see evaluation form)
2. Quiz on lecture material
3. Faculty to evaluate strengths and weaknesses of this module, with suggestions for improvement

Module 4: Loss, Grief, and Bereavement

PRE-CLASS ASSIGNMENT

Consult module bibliography and instructional resources for possible pre-class reading and/or assignments.

LEARNING OBJECTIVES

Upon completion of this module, students will be able to:

- Identify different bereavement situations
- Describe manifestations of uncomplicated responses to loss
- Describe differences in grieving for diverse populations
- Describe several social work interventions to aid grieving clients

LECTURE OUTLINE

1. Introduction: Why is it important for social work students to learn about loss, grief, and bereavement? Loss permeates human experience, and social workers are likely to find issues of grief and loss in any and all practice settings.
2. Definitions
    a. Mourning
    b. Grief
    c. Bereavement
3. Possible bereavement situations / special considerations
    a. Anticipatory grief
    b. Developmental considerations
    c. Modes of death
    d. Special issues for people who have experienced the sudden death of a loved one
4. Grief responses: Theories and models
    a. The grief cycle: Reaction, resistance, reality, resignation, reorganization
    b. Tasks of mourning
    c. Development landmarks and tasks at end of life
    d. Critique of models and state theories
    e. Stroebe and Schut's dual-processing model
    f. Cultural differences in mourning
    g. Complicated grief reactions

5. Helping clients through grief and loss
   a. What could you say to someone who is grieving?
   b. What should you *not* say?
   c. What do people who are grieving need?
   d. Some specific social work interventions with grieving people

INSTRUCTIONAL RESOURCES

Small Group Activities

Assign students in small groups a nonmedical practice setting (e.g., child protection, school, foster care, camp, adoption agency, senior services, criminal justice/corrections, emergency services, basic needs agencies). Then ask each group to discuss this question: In what ways might loss and grief arise for social work clients in this setting? Consider possible scenarios for an individual, a group, a family, the agency, or the community it serves. Students should write down all possibilities and be prepared to share at least two situations with the class.

In small groups, review a case study (or several different ones) with diversity variables (age, religion, ethnicity) and have students answer questions such as, Who else needs to know about your work with this client/family? What is the future plan with this client? Have students present their answers to the class.

Discussion Questions

1. Why is it important for social workers in different practice settings to know the signs of grieving and bereavement?
2. What are some of the factors or predictors that can influence how a person grieves a loss?

Assignments

1. Have students write a condolence letter and/or collect sample ones from friends and family. Alternatively, have students bring in sympathy cards. Evaluate the effectiveness of these messages. What kind of messages are likely to be helpful? Harmful?
2. Visit a hospice program to request a copy of the program's psychosocial assessment forms.
3. Both the book and the film versions of *Ordinary People* provide an excellent lens through which to assess the grief process. The assessment format can be provided by the instructor; William Worden provides excellent assessment models that can be used.

BIBLIOGRAPHY

Bern-Klug, M. (2004). The ambiguous dying syndrome. *Health and Social Work, 29,* 55–65.

Bern-Klug, M., Ekerdt, D. J., & Wilkinson, D. S. (1999). What families know about funeral-related costs: Implications for social work practice. *Health and Social Work, 24*(2), 128–137.

Brandsen, C. K. (2005). Social work and end-of-life care: Reviewing the past and moving forward. *Journal of Social Work in End-of-Life and Palliative Care, 1*(2), 45–70.

Breitbart, W., Rosenfeld, B., Pessin, H., Kaim, M., Funesti-Esch, J., Galietta, M., et al. (2000). Depression, hopelessness, and desire for hastened death in terminally ill patients with cancer. *Journal of the American Medical Association, 284*(22), 2907–2911.

Collins, C., Liken, M., King, S., & Kokinakis, K. (1993). Loss and grief among family caregivers of relatives with dementia. *Qualitative Health Research, 3*(2), 236–253.

Fauri, D. P., Ettner, B., & Kovacs, P. J. (2000). Bereavement services in acute care settings. *Death Studies, 24*(1), 51–64.

Gray, S. W., Zide, M. R., & Wilker, H. (2000). Using the solution focused brief therapy model with bereavement groups in rural communities: Resiliency at its best. *Hospice Journal, 15,* 13–30.

Lister, L. (1991). Men and grief: A review of research. *Smith College Studies in Social Work, 61*(3), 220–235.

Lord, B., & Pockett, R. (1998). Perceptions of social work intervention with bereaved clients: Some implications for hospital social work practice. *Social Work in Health Care, 27*(1), 51–66.

Murphy, K., Hanrahan, P., & Luchins, D. (1997). A survey of grief and bereavement in nursing homes: The importance of hospice grief and bereavement for the end-stage Alzheimer's disease patient and family. *Journal of the American Geriatrics Society, 49*(9), 1104–1107.

Papadatou, D. (1997). Training health professionals in caring for dying children and grieving families. *Death Studies, 21,* 575–600.

Pauw, M. (1991). The social worker's role with a fetal demise and stillbirth. *Health and Social Work, 16,* 291–297.

Roberts, C. S., Baile, W. F., & Bassett, J. D. (1999). When the care giver needs care. *Social Work in Health Care, 30*(2), 65–80.

Walker, R. J., Pomeroy, E. C., & McNeil, J. S. (1996). Anticipatory grief and AIDS: Strategies for intervening with caregivers. *Health and Social Work, 21*(1), 49–57.

Walsh-Burke, K. (2000). Matching bereavement services to level of need. *Hospice Journal, 15,* 77–86.

Wells, P. J. (1993). Preparing for sudden death: Social work in the emergency room. *Social Work, 38,* 339–342.

Werth, J. L. (1999). The role of the mental health professional in helping significant others of persons who are assisted in death. *Death Studies, 23*(3), 239–255.

WEBLIOGRAPHY

Bereavement and Medical Emergency Travelers: http://www.bereavementair.com

Bereavement Hospitality Services: http://www.bereavetravel.com

End of Life / Palliative Resource Education Center: www.eperc.mcw.edu

EVALUATION

1. Self-evaluation (have students rank themselves on module learning objectives; see evaluation form)
2. Quiz on lecture material
3. Faculty to evaluate strengths and weaknesses of this module, with suggestions for improvement

Module 5: The Intersection of Ethics, Practice, and Policy in End-of-Life Care

PRE-CLASS ASSIGNMENT

Consult module bibliography and instructional resources for possible pre-class reading and/or assignments.

LEARNING OBJECTIVES

Upon completion of this module, students will:

- Understand the distinctions between values and ethics, the primary strands of ethical thinking throughout history in the Western world, and what constitutes an ethical dilemma
- Be familiar with relevant sections of the NASW *Code of Ethics* and NASW policy statements with respect to end-of-life care
- Have a basic understanding of autonomy, beneficence, non-maleficence, and justice
- Be familiar with landmark ethical cases with respect to end-of-life care
- Be able to recognize the ethical arenas where social workers are likely to be involved and are expected to have expertise
- Be able to use a decision-making model for resolving ethical dilemmas with respect to end-of-life issues
- Be able to demonstrate critical thinking skills with respect to unjust practice standards and policies in end-of-life care

INSTRUCTIONAL RESOURCES

Small Group Activities and Exercises

Have students complete sections 1 and 2 of the Five Wishes document. Ask them to pay attention to the difficult decision-making points as they do this. Discuss.

Present students with the case addressed in "An Alert and Incompetent Self: The Irrelevance of Advance Directives" (in the *Hasitngs Center Report*), and follow it up with questions to consider. Many of the case studies in the *Hastings Center Report* can be adapted for small group discussion on various ethical principles. Each case study is followed by differing responses from at least two experts. After students have grappled with the complexity of a case, they usually find it interesting to read the responses of the experts.

Films

Dax's Case: Who Should Decide. This is an excellent film to use to demonstrate the tensions between various ethical principles.

Who Owns My Life? The Sue Rodriguez Story. This film is useful for discussing the issues involved in physician-assisted suicide.

A Choice for K'aila: May Parents Refuse a Transplant for Their Child? This film is useful for highlighting tensions between the values of Western medicine and traditional Native American beliefs with respect to transplantation, as well as the question of who (society or parents) should be responsible for aggressive medical treatment of infants.

On Being Old, Black, and Poor. This film tells the story of an elderly couple living in Chicago and the concerns of many professionals (health care, adult protection, community services) about whether and how the couple can live in their own apartment when both are in failing health. This is a powerful depiction of the self-determination versus best interest standards for end-of-life care.

Speakers

If one is available, invite a social worker who sits on the institutional ethics committee of an acute care hospital or nursing home facility. Ask him or her to talk about his or her role on this committee and how challenging ethical decisions are made. Or invite a social worker who works in a nursing home or home care context. Ask the social worker to discuss the everyday ethical dilemmas encountered in his or her work, and how such dilemmas are resolved.

Field Trips

Visit an assisted breathing center or a residential facility for people with Alzheimer's. Talk with staff, family, and patients about the ethical dilemmas they encounter on a daily basis. If staff and patients are willing, discuss how they know when "enough is enough." Often these facilities employ social workers as part of the interdisciplinary team. If one is available, talk with the social worker about his or her role, the ethical dilemmas encountered, and how decisions are made in these dilemmas. Note: The benefit to visiting facilities like these is that students are able to meet the residents whose lives are being discussed. Seeing these people in the flesh makes the gravity of decision making more real and more complex.

BIBLIOGRAPHY

Adler, S. S. (1989). Truth telling to the terminally ill: Neglected role of the social worker. *Social Work, 34*(2), 158–160.

Brandsen, C. K. (2005). Social work and end-of-life care: Reviewing the past and moving forward. *Journal of Social Work in End-of-Life and Palliative Care, 1*(2), 45–70.

Callahan, J. (1994). The ethics of assisted suicide. *Health and Social Work, 19*(4), 237–244.

Casarett, D. J., Karlawish, J. H. T., & Byock, I. (2002). Advocacy and activism: Missing pieces in the quest to improve end-of-life care. *Journal of Palliative Medicine, 5,* 3–12.

Csikai, E. L. (1999). Euthanasia and assisted suicide: Issues for social work practice. *Journal of Gerontological Social Work, 31*(3/4), 49–63.

Csikai, E. L. (1999). Hospital social worker attitudes toward euthanasia and assisted suicide. *Social Work in Health Care, 30*(1), 57–73.

Csikai, E. L. (1999). The role of values and experience in determining social workers' attitudes toward euthanasia and assisted suicide. *Social Work in Health Care, 30*(1), 75–95.

Csikai, E. L. (2002). The state of hospice ethics committees and the social work role. *Omega: Journal of Death and Dying, 45,* 261–275.

Csikai, E. L. (2004). Social workers' participation in the resolution of ethical dilemmas in hospice care. *Health and Social Work, 29,* 67–76.

Csikai, E. L., & Bass, K. (2000). Health care social workers' views of ethical issues, practice, and policy in end-of-life care. *Social Work in Health Care, 32*(2), 1–22.

Galambos, C. M. (1998). Preserving end-of-life autonomy: The Patient Self-Determination Act and the Uniform Health Care Decisions Act. *Health and Social Work, 23*(4), 275–281.

Gordon, M. (2002). Ethical challenges in end-of-life therapies in the elderly. *Drugs and Aging, 19,* 321–329.

Gunter-Hunt, G., Mahoney, J. E., & Sieger, C. E. (2002). A comparison of state advance directive documents. *The Gerontologist, 42,* 51–60.

Gwyther, L. P., Altilio, T., Blacker, S., Christ, G., Csikai, E. L., Hooyman, N., et al. (2005). Social work competencies in palliative and end-of-life care. *Journal of Social Work in End-of-Life and Palliative Care, 1,* 87–120.

Kadushin, G., & Egan, M. (2001). Ethical dilemmas in home health care: A social work perspective. *Health and Social Work, 26,* 136–149.

Keigher, S. (1994). Patient rights and dying: Policy restraint and the states. *Health and Social Work, 19*(4), 298–303.

Leichtentritt, R. D., & Rettig, K. D. (2001). Values underlying end-of-life decisions: A qualitative approach. *Health and Social Work, 26,* 150–159.

Manetta, A. A., & Wells, J. G. (2001). Ethical issues in the social worker's role in physician-assisted suicide. *Health and Social Work, 26,* 160–166.

Mezey, M., Mitty, E., Rappaport, M., & Ramsey, G. (1997). Implementation of the Patient Self-Determination Act (PSDA) in nursing homes in New York City. *Journal of the American Geriatrics Society, 45*(1), 43–49.

Miller, P. J. (2000). Life after death with dignity: The Oregon experience. *Social Work, 45,* 263–271.

Miller, P. J., Hedlund, S. C., & Murphy, K. A. (1998). Social work assessment at end of life: Practice guidelines for suicide and the terminally ill. *Social Work in Health Care, 26*(4), 23–26.

Miller, P. J., Mesler, M. A., & Eggman, S. T. (2002). Take some time to look inside their hearts: Hospice social workers contemplate physician assisted suicide. *Social Work in Health Care, 35*(3), 53–64.

National Association of Social Workers. (2000). *Social work speaks: NASW policy statements.* Washington, DC: NASW Press.

Ogden, R. D., & Young, M. G. (2003). Washington State social workers' attitudes toward voluntary euthanasia and assisted suicide. *Social Work in Health Care, 37*(2), 43–70.

Osman, H., & Perlin, T. M. (1994). Patient self-determination and the artificial prolongation of life. *Health and Social Work, 19*(4), 245–252.

Roff, S. (2001). Analyzing end-of-life care legislation: A social work perspective. *Social Work in Health Care, 33,* 51–68.

Silverman, E. (1992). Hospital bioethics: A beginning knowledge base for the neonatal social worker. *Social Work, 37,* 150–154.

Werth, J. L. (2002). Legal and ethical considerations for mental health professionals related to end-of-life care and decision making. *American Behavioral Scientist, 46,* 373–383.

Werth, J. L., & Blevins, D. (2002). Public policy and end-of-life care. *American Behavioral Scientist, 46,* 401–417.

Werth, J. L., Blevins, D., Toussaint, K. L., & Durham, M. R. (2002). The influence of cultural diversity on end-of-life care and decisions. *American Behavioral Scientist, 46,* 204–219.

Wesley, C. A. (1996). Social work and end-of-life decisions: Self-determination and the common good. *Health and Social Work, 21*(2), 115–121.

EVALUATION

1. Self-evaluation (have students rank themselves on module learning objectives; see evaluation form)
2. Quiz on lecture material
3. Faculty to evaluate strengths and weaknesses of this module, with suggestions for improvement

Student Self-Evaluation: Module 1

How well did this class increase your ability to:	Very well	Fairly well	Not well at all
Define end of life?			
Understand the demographics, trends and major social issues for death and dying?			
Identify different services available to people at the end of their lives?			
Identify the relationship of end-of-life issues to various social work practice settings?			
Describe several social policy issues in death and dying?			

Student Self-Evaluation: Module 2

How well did this class increase your ability to:	Very well	Fairly well	Not well at all
Explore your own values about death and dying to assess readiness to begin practice?			
Recognize the richness and value in the experiences of loss and dying?			
Gain personal and professional confidence regarding end-of-life practice?			
Describe two strategies for self-care?			

Student Self-Evaluation: Module 3

How well did this class increase your ability to:	Very well	Fairly well	Not well at all
Understand the physiological process of dying?			
Describe categories in a complete social assessment of dying persons and their families?			
Understand a range of psycho-social and case management interventions commonly needed by persons at the end of life and their loved ones?			
Recognize cultural differences in the dying experience?			

Student Self-Evaluation: Module 4

How well did this class increase your ability to:	Very well	Fairly well	Not well at all
Identify different bereavement situations?			
Describe manifestations of uncomplicated responses to loss?			
Describe differences in grieving for diverse populations?			
Describe several interventions to aid grieving clients?			

Student Self-Evaluation: Module 5

On a scale from 1 to 5 (1 indicating that you have learned nothing of value with respect to this topic, and 5 indicating that you have learned a great deal), please rank your learning.

_____ I understand the distinctions between values and ethics.

_____ I have a basic understanding of the primary strands of ethical thinking.

_____ I understand what constitutes an ethical dilemma.

_____ I am familiar with relevant sections of the NASW *Code of Ethics*.

_____ I am familiar with relevant social work policy statements.

_____ I have a basic understanding of autonomy, beneficence, nonmaleficence, and justice.

_____ I am familiar with landmark ethical cases with respect to end-of-life care.

_____ I recognize the ethical arenas where social workers are likely to be involved and are expected to have expertise.

_____ I am able to use a decision-making model for resolving ethical dilemmas with respect to end-of-life issues.

_____ I have a basic understanding of unjust practice standards and policies in end-of-life care.

BIBLIOGRAPHY

Abramson, J. S., & Mizrahi, T. (1996). When social workers and physicians collaborate: Positive and negative interdisciplinary experiences. *Social Work, 41,* 270–281.

Adler, S. S. (1989). Truth telling to the terminally ill: Neglected role of the social worker. *Social Work, 34*(2), 158–160.

Amar, D. F. (1994). The role of the hospice social worker in the nursing home setting. *American Journal of Hospice and Palliative Care, 11*(3), 18–22.

Arnold, E. M. (2004). Factors that influence consideration of hastening death among people with life-threatening illnesses. *Health and Social Work, 29,* 17–26.

Back, A. (2000). Communication between professions: Doctors are from Mars, social workers are from Venus. *Journal of Palliative Medicine, 3*(2), 221–222.

Back, A. L., Wallace, J. I., Starks, H. E., & Pearlman, R. A. (1996). Physician-assisted suicide and euthanasia in Washington State: Patient requests and physician responses. *Journal of the American Medical Association, 275*(12), 919–925.

Bailly, D. J., & DePoy, E. (1995). Older people's responses to education about advance directives. *Health and Social Work, 20*(3), 223–228.

Baker, M. E. (2000). Knowledge and attitudes of health care social workers regarding advance directives. *Social Work in Health Care, 32,* 61–74.

Becker, J. E. (2004). Oncology social workers' attitudes toward hospice care and referral behavior. *Health and Social Work, 29,* 36–45.

Bern-Klug, M. (2004). The ambiguous dying syndrome. *Health and Social Work, 29,* 55–65.

Bern-Klug, M., Ekerdt, D. J., & Wilkinson, D. S. (1999). What families know about funeral-related costs: Implications for social work practice. *Health and Social Work, 24*(2), 128–137.

Bern-Klug, M., Gessert, C., & Forbes, S. (2001). The need to revise assumptions about the end of life: Implications for social work practice. *Health and Social Work, 26*(1), 38–48.

Botsford, A. L. (2000). Integrating end-of-life care into services for people with an intellectual disability. *Social Work in Health Care, 31*(1), 35–48.

Brandsen, C. K. (2005). Social work and end-of-life care: Reviewing the past and moving forward. *Journal of Social Work in End-of-Life and Palliative Care, 1*(2), 45–70.

Breitbart, W., Rosenfeld, B., Pessin, H., Kaim, M., Funesti-Esch, J., Galietta, M., et al. (2000). Depression, hopelessness, and desire for hastened death in terminally ill patients with cancer. *Journal of the American Medical Association, 284*(22), 2907–2911.

Broome, B. J., DeTurk, S., Kristjansdottir, E. S., Kanasta, T., & Ganesan, P. (2002). Giving voice to diversity: An interactive approach to conflict management and decision-making in culturally diverse work environments. *Journal of Business and Management, 8,* 239–264.

Brown, M. (1999). Psychosocial functions and training needs of social workers in nursing homes: A survey. *Continuum, 19*(1), 7–13.

Callahan, J. (1994). The ethics of assisted suicide. *Health and Social Work, 19*(4), 237–244.

Care at the End of Life. (2000). *Best practice series: Innovative practice in social work.* Philadelphia: Society for Social Work Leadership in Health Care.

Casarett, D. J., Karlawish, J. H. T., & Byock, I. (2002). Advocacy and activism: Missing pieces in the quest to improve end-of-life care. *Journal of Palliative Medicine, 5,* 3–12.

Chichin, E. R., Ferster, L., & Gordon, N. (1994). Planning for the end of life with the home care client. *Journal of Gerontological Social Work, 22*(1/2), 147–159.

Christ, G., & Blacker, S. (2005). Setting an agenda for social work in end-of-life care: An overview of leadership and organizational initiatives. *Journal of Social Work in End-of-Life and Palliative Care, 1*(1), 9–17.

Christ, G., & Sormanti M. (1999). Advancing social work practice in end-of-life care. *Social Work in Health Care, 30*(2), 81–99.

Chung, K. (1993). Brief social work intervention in the hospice setting: Person-centered work and crisis intervention synthesized and distilled. *Palliative Medicine, 7*(1), 59–62.

Cochran, D. L. (1999). Advance elder care decision making: A model of family planning. *Journal of Gerontological Social Work, 32*(2), 53–64.

Collins, C., Liken, M., King, S., & Kokinakis, K. (1993). Loss and grief among family caregivers of relatives with dementia. *Qualitative Health Research, 3*(2), 236–253.

Coluzzi, P. H., Grant, M., Doroshow, J. H., Rhiner, M., Ferrell, B., & Rivera, L. (1995).

Survey of the provision of supportive care services at National Cancer Institute-designated cancer centers. *Journal of Clinical Oncology, 13*(3), 756–764.

Connor, S. R., Egan, K. A., Kwilosz, D. M., Larson, D. G., & Reese, D. J. (2002). Interdisciplinary approaches to assisting with end-of-life care and decision making. *American Behavioral Scientist, 46,* 340–356.

Cowles, L. A., & Lefcowitz, M. J. (1992). Interdisciplinary expectations of the medical social worker in the hospital setting. *Health and Social Work, 17,* 57–65.

Csikai, E. L. (1999). Euthanasia and assisted suicide: Issues for social work practice. *Journal of Gerontological Social Work, 31*(3/4), 49–63.

Csikai, E. L. (1999). Hospital social worker attitudes toward euthanasia and assisted suicide. *Social Work in Health Care, 30*(1), 57–73.

Csikai, E. L. (1999). The role of values and experience in determining social workers' attitudes toward euthanasia and assisted suicide. *Social Work in Health Care, 30*(1), 75–95.

Csikai, E. L. (2002). The state of hospice ethics committees and the social work role. *Omega: Journal of Death and Dying, 45,* 261–275.

Csikai, E. L. (2004). Social workers' participation in the resolution of ethical dilemmas in hospice care. *Health and Social Work, 29,* 67–76.

Csikai, E. L., & Bass, K. (2000). Health care social workers' views of ethical issues, practice, and policy in end-of-life care. *Social Work in Health Care, 32*(2), 1–22.

Csikai, E. L., & Manetta, A. A. (2002). Preventing unnecessary deaths among older adults: A call to action for social workers. *Journal of Gerontological Social Work, 38,* 85–97.

Csikai, E. L., & Raymer, M. (2004). *Health care social workers' educational needs in end-of-life care.* Unpublished manuscript.

Dane, B. O., & Miller, S. O. (1990). AIDS and dying: The teaching challenge. *Journal of Teaching in Social Work, 4*(1), 85–100.

Davidson, K. W., & Foster, Z. (1995). Social work with dying and bereaved clients: Helping the workers. *Social Work in Health Care, 21*(4), 1–16.

Davitt, J. K., & Kaye, L. W. (1996). Supporting patient autonomy: Decision making in home health care. *Social Work, 41*(1), 41–50.

Dickinson, G. E., Sumner, E. D., & Frederick, L. M. (1992). Death education in selected health professions. *Death Studies, 16,* 281–289.

Dunbar, H. T., Mueller, C. W., & Medina, C. (1998). Psychological and spiritual growth in women living with HIV. *Social Work, 43*(2).

Dungan, S. S., Jaquay, T. R., Rezink, K. A., & Sands, E. A. (1995). Pediatric critical care social work: Clinical practice with parents of critically ill children. *Social Work in Health Care, 21*(1), 69–80.

Egan, M., & Kadushin, G. (1999). The social worker in the emerging field of home care: Professional activities and ethical concerns. *Health and Social Work, 24*(1), 43–55.

Fauri, D. P., Ettner, B., & Kovacs, P. J. (2000). Bereavement services in acute care settings. *Death Studies, 24*(1), 51–64.

Finucane, T. E. (1999). How gravely ill becomes dying: A key to end-of-life care. *Journal of the American Medical Association, 282*(17), 1670–1672.

Foster, A., & Davidson, K. (1995). Satisfactions and stresses for the social worker. In I. Corless, B. B. Germino, & M. A. Pittman-Lindman (Eds.), *Dying, death, and bereavement: A challenge for living* (pp. 285–300). Boston: Jones and Bartlett.

Foster, L. W., & McLellan, L. J. (2002). Translating psychosocial insight into ethical discussions supportive of families in end-of-life decision making. *Social Work in Health Care, 35,* 37–51.

Galambos, C. M. (1998). Preserving end-of-life autonomy: The Patient Self-Determination Act and the Uniform Health Care Decisions Act. *Health and Social Work, 23*(4), 275–281.

Glajchen, M., Blum, D., & Calder, K. (1995). Cancer pain management and the role of social work: Barriers and interventions. *Health and Social Work, 20*(3), 200–206.

Gordon, M. (2002). Ethical challenges in end-of-life therapies in the elderly. *Drugs and Aging, 19,* 321–329.

Gray, S. W., Zide, M. R., & Wilker, H. (2000). Using the solution focused brief therapy model with bereavement groups in rural communities: Resiliency at its best. *Hospice Journal, 15,* 13–30.

Gunter-Hunt, G., Mahoney, J. E., & Sieger, C. E. (2002). A comparison of state advance directive documents. *The Gerontologist, 42,* 51–60.

Gwyther, L. P., Altilio, T., Blacker, S., Christ, G., Csikai, E. L., Hooyman, N., et al. (2005). Social work competencies in palliative and end-of-life care. *Journal of Social Work in End-of-Life and Palliative Care, 1,* 87–120.

Hobart, K. R. (2001). Death and dying and the social work role. *Journal of Gerontological Social Work, 36,* 181–192.

Hoffman, M. K. (1994). Use of advance directives: A social work perspective on the myth versus the reality. *Death Studies, 18*(3), 229–241.

Itzhaky, H., & Lipschitz-Elhawi, R. (2004). Hope as a strategy in supervising social workers of terminally ill patients. *Health and Social Work, 29,* 46–54.

Kadushin, G., & Egan, M. (2001). Ethical dilemmas in home health care: A social work perspective. *Health and Social Work, 26,* 136–149.

Keigher, S. (1994). Patient rights and dying: Policy restraint and the states. *Health and Social Work, 19*(4), 298–303.

Kinsella, G., Cooper, B., Picton, C., & Murtagh, D. (2000). Factors influencing outcomes for family caregivers of persons receiving palliative care: Toward an integrated model. *Journal of Palliative Care, 16*(3), 46–54.

Knebel, A., & Buckwalter, K. C. (2002). End-of-life research: Focus on older populations. *The Gerontologist, 42* (Special edition), 4–9.

Kovacs, P. J., & Bronstein, L. R. (1999). Preparation for oncology settings: What hospice social workers say they need. *Health and Social Work, 24*(1), 57–64.

Kramer, B. J. (1998). Preparing social workers for the inevitable: A preliminary investigation of a course on grief, death, and loss. *Journal of Social Work Education, 34,* 211–227.

Kramer, B. J., Christ, G. H., Francoeur, R. B., & Bern-Klug, M. (2004). *A national agenda for social work research in palliative and end-of-life care.* Unpublished manuscript.

Kramer, B. J., Pacourek, L., & Hovland-Scafe, C. (2003). Analysis of end-of-life content in social work textbooks. *Journal of Social Work Education, 39,* 299–320.

Kristjanson, L., Dudgeon, D., Nelson, F., Henteleff, P., & Balneaves, L. (1997). Evaluation of an interdisciplinary training program in palliative care: Addressing the needs of rural and northern communities. *Journal of Palliative Care, 13*(3), 5–12.

Kulys, R., & Davis, M. A. (1986). An analysis of social services in hospices. *Social Work, 31*(6), 448–456.

Landau, R. (1996). Preparing for sudden death or organ donation: An ethical dilemma in social work. *International Social Work, 39,* 431.

Leichtentritt, R. D., & Rettig, K. D. (2001). Values underlying end-of-life decisions: A qualitative approach. *Health and Social Work, 26,* 150–159.

Lethem, W. (1999). Nursing homes deliver palliative care. *Nursing Times, 3*(95), 55.

Lister, L. (1991). Men and grief: A review of research. *Smith College Studies in Social Work, 61*(3), 220–235.

Lord, B., & Pockett, R. (1998). Perceptions of social work intervention with bereaved clients: Some implications for hospital social work practice. *Social Work in Health Care, 27*(1), 51–66.

Loscalzo, M. L., & Bucher, J. A. (1999). The COPE model: Its clinical usefulness in solving pain-related problems. *Journal of Psychosocial Oncology, 16*(3/4), 93–117.

Lunney, J. R., Foley, K. M., Smith, T. J., & Gelband, H. (Eds.). (2003). *Describing death in America.* Washington, DC: National Academy Press.

Luptak, M. (2004). Social work and end-of-life care for older people: A historical perspective. *Health and Social Work, 29,* 7–15.

MacDonald, D. (1991). Hospice social work: A search for identity. *Health and Social Work, 16*(4), 274–280.

Manetta, A. A., & Wells, J. G. (2001). Ethical issues in the social worker's role in physician-assisted suicide. *Health and Social Work, 26,* 160–166.

McDaniel, B. A. (1989). A group work experience with mentally retarded adults on the issues of death and dying. *Journal of Gerontological Social Work, 13*(3/4), 187–191.

Mesler, M. A. (1994–1995). The philosophy and practice of patient control in hospice: The dynamics of autonomy versus paternalism. *Omega: Journal of Death and Dying, 30*(3), 173–189.

Mesler, M. A. (1995). Negotiating life for the dying: Hospice and the strategy of tactical socialization. *Death Studies, 19,* 235–255.

Mezey, M., Mitty, E., Rappaport, M., & Ramsey, G. (1997). Implementation of the Patient Self-Determination Act (PSDA) in nursing homes in New York City. *Journal of the American Geriatrics Society, 45*(1), 43–49.

Miller, P. J. (2000). Life after death with dignity: The Oregon experience. *Social Work, 45,* 263–271.

Miller, P. J., Hedlund, S. C., & Murphy, K. A. (1998). Social work assessment at end of life: Practice guidelines for suicide and the terminally ill. *Social Work in Health Care, 26*(4), 23–26.

Miller, P. J., Mesler, M. A., & Eggman, S. T. (2002). Take some time to look inside their hearts: Hospice social workers contemplate physician assisted suicide. *Social Work in Health Care, 35*(3), 53–64.

Mizrahi, T., & Abramson, J. (1985). Sources of strain between physicians and social workers: Implications for social workers in health care settings. *Social Work in Health Care, 10*(3), 33–51.

Monroe, B. (1994). Role of the social worker in palliative care. *Annals of the Academy of Medicine, Singapore, 23*(2), 252–255.

Moynihan, R., Christ, G., & Silver L. G. (1988). AIDS and terminal illness. *Social Casework, 69*(6), 380–387.

Mularski, R. A., Bascom, P., & Osborne, M. L. (2001). Educational agendas for interdisciplinary end-of-life curricula. *Critical Care Medicine, 29,* 16–23.

Murphy, K., Hanrahan, P., & Luchins, D. (1997). A survey of grief and bereavement in nursing homes: The importance of hospice grief and bereavement for the end-stage Alzheimer's disease patient and family. *Journal of the American Geriatrics Society, 49*(9), 1104–1107.

Nardi, D. A., Ornelas, F., Wright, M., & Crispell, R. (2001). Clergy and social workers' attitudes toward death and palliative care in an acute care setting. *International Journal of Palliative Nursing, 7,* 30–36.

National Association of Social Workers. (2000). *Social work speaks: NASW policy statements.* Washington, DC: NASW Press.

National Consensus Project for Quality Palliative Care. (2004). *Clinical practice guidelines for quality palliative care.* Retrieved July 15, 2004, from http://www.nationalconsensusproject.org

Neron, C. (1996). Euthanasia, assisted suicide and HIV/AIDS: Implications for social work. *The Social Worker, 64*(4), 129–136.

Neuman, K., & Wade, L. (1999). Advance directives: The experience of health care professionals across the continuum of care. *Social Work in Health Care, 28*(3), 39–54.

Nicholson, B. L., & Matross, G. N. (1989). Facing reduced decision-making capacity in health care: Method for maintaining client self-determination. *Social Work, 34*(3), 234–238.

Ogden, R. D., & Young, M. G. (1998). Euthanasia and assisted suicide: A survey of registered social workers in British Columbia. *British Journal of Social Work, 28*(2), 161–175.

Ogden, R. D., & Young, M. G. (2003). Washington State social workers' attitudes toward voluntary euthanasia and assisted suicide. *Social Work in Health Care, 37*(2), 43–70.

Osman, H., & Perlin, T. M. (1994). Patient self-determination and the artificial prolongation of life. *Health and Social Work, 19*(4), 245–252.

Papadatou, D. (1997). Training health professionals in caring for dying children and grieving families. *Death Studies, 21,* 575–600.

Pauw, M. (1991). The social worker's role with a fetal demise and stillbirth. *Health and Social Work, 16,* 291–297.

Quig, L. (1989). The role of the hospice social worker. *American Journal of Hospice Care, 6*(4), 22–23.

Quinn, A. (1998). Learning from palliative care: Concepts to underpin the transfer of knowledge from specialist palliative care to mainstream social work settings. *Social Work Education, 17*(1), 9–20.

Reese, D. J., Ahern, R. E., Nair, S., O'Faire, J. D., & Warren, C. (1999). Hospice access and use by African Americans: Addressing cultural and institutional barriers through participatory action research. *Social Work, 44*(6), 549–559.

Reese, D. J., & Brown, D. R. (1997). Psychosocial and spiritual care in hospice: Differences between nursing, social work, and clergy. *Hospice Journal, 12*(1), 29–41.

Reese, D. J., & Raymer, M. (2004). Relationships between social work involvement and hospice outcomes: Results of the national hospice social work survey. *Social Work, 49,* 415–422.

Reese, D. J., & Sontag, M. (2001). Successful interprofessional collaboration on the hospice team. *Health and Social Work, 26,* 167–175.

Remsen, M. F. (1993). The role of the nursing home social worker in terminal care. *Journal of Gerontological Social Work, 19*(3/4), 193–205.

Rice, J. R., Hicks, P. B., & Wiehe, V. (2000). Life care planning: A role for social workers. *Social Work in Health Care, 31*(1), 85–94.

Roberts, C. S. (1989). Conflicting professional values in social work and medicine. *Health and Social Work, 14*(3), 211–218.

Roberts, C. S., Baile, W. F., & Bassett, J. D. (1999). When the care giver needs care. *Social Work in Health Care, 30*(2), 65–80.

Roff, S. (2001). Analyzing end-of-life care legislation: A social work perspective. *Social Work in Health Care, 33,* 51–68.

Rosen, A., & O'Neill, J. (1998). *Social work roles and opportunities in advanced directives and health care decision-making*. Retrieved March 1998 from http://www.socialworkers.org/practice/aging/advdirct.asp

Rusnack, B., Schaefer, S. M., & Moxley, D. (1988). "Safe passage": Social work roles and functions in hospice care. *Social Work in Health Care, 13*(3), 3–19.

Rusnack, B., Schaefer, S. M., & Moxley, D. (1990). Hospice: Social work's response to a new form of social caring. *Social Work in Health Care, 15,* 95–119.

Sakadakis, V., Bonar, R., & Maclean, M. J. (1987). The role of the social worker in terminal care with institutionalized elderly people. *Journal of Palliative Care, 3*(2), 19–25.

Schroeder, M. R. (1997). Guidelines for care of the dying patient: An interdisciplinary effort. *Continuum, 17*(1), 3–10.

Shafer, D. (1993). Ethical dilemmas for the social worker involved in life and death decision making. *Jewish Social Work Forum, 29,* 52–67.

Sheldon, F. M. (2000). Dimensions of the role of the social worker in palliative care. *Palliative Medicine, 14*(6), 491–498.

Sieppert, J. D. (1996). Attitudes toward and knowledge of chronic pain: A survey of medical social workers. *Health and Social Work, 21*(2), 122–130.

Silverman, E. (1992). Hospital bioethics: A beginning knowledge base for the neonatal social worker. *Social Work, 37,* 150–154.

Singer, P. A., Martin, D. K., & Kelner, M. (1999). Quality-of-life care: Patients' perspectives. *Journal of the American Medical Association, 281*(2), 163–168.

Skobel, S. W., Cullom, B. A., & Showalter, S. E. (1997). When a nurse is not enough: Why the hospice interdisciplinary team may be a nurse's best gift. *American Journal of Hospice and Palliative Care, 14*(4), 201–204.

Smith, E. D. (1995). Addressing the psycho-spiritual distress of death as reality: A transpersonal approach. *Social Work, 40*(3), 402–413.

Smith, S. H. (1999). "Now that Mom is in the Lord's arms, I just have to live the way she taught me": Reflections on an elderly, African American mother's death. *Journal of Gerontological Social Work, 32*(2), 41–51.

Smokowski, P. R., & Wodarski, J. S. (1996). Euthanasia and physician assisted suicide: A social work update. *Social Work in Health Care, 23*(1), 53–65.

Sormanti, M. (1994). Fieldwork instruction in oncology social work: Supervisory issues. *Journal of Psychosocial Oncology, 12,* 73–87.

Soskis, C. W. (1997). End-of-life decisions in the home care setting. *Social Work in Health Care, 25*(1/2), 107–116.

Stahl, S. (2000). *End-of-life research conference proposal. Working paper to establish a National Institute on Aging research agenda in end-of-life care*. Bethesda, MD: National Institute on Aging / National Institutes of Health.

Stein, G. L. (2004). Improving our care at life's end: Making a difference. *Health and Social Work, 29,* 77–79.

Stoesen, L. (2002). Role in end-of-life care examined. *NASW News, 47*(5), 4.

Storey, P. (1994). Social workers and volunteers at different stages of palliative care. *American Journal of Hospice and Palliative Care, 11*(2), 5–7.

Taylor-Brown, S., Teeter, J. A., & Blackburn, E. (1998). Parental loss due to HIV: Caring for children as a community issue—the Rochester, New York experience. *Child Welfare, 77*(2), 137–160.

Thompson, M., Rose, C., Wainwright, W., Mattar, L., & Scanlan, M. (2001). Activities of counselors in a hospice/palliative care environment. *Journal of Palliative Care, 17,* 229–235.

Vachon, M. L. S. (1986). Myths and realities in palliative/hospice care. *Hospice Journal, 2*(1), 63–79.

Van Bloch, L. (1996). Breaking the bad news when sudden death occurs. *Social Work in Health Care, 23*(4), 91–97.

Van Loon, R. A. (1999). Desire to die in terminally ill people: A framework for assessment and intervention. *Health and Social Work, 24*(4), 260–268.

Walker, R. J., Pomeroy, E. C., & McNeil, J. S. (1994). Anticipatory grief and Alzheimer's disease: Strategies for intervention. *Journal of Gerontological Social Work, 22*(3/4), 21–39.

Walker, R. J., Pomeroy, E. C., & McNeil, J. S. (1996). Anticipatory grief and AIDS: Strategies for intervening with caregivers. *Health and Social Work, 21*(1), 49–57.

Walsh-Burke, K. (2000). Matching bereavement services to level of need. *Hospice Journal, 15,* 77–86.

Wells, P. J. (1993). Preparing for sudden death: Social work in the emergency room. *Social Work, 38,* 339–342.

Werner, P., Carmel, S., & Ziedenberg, H. (2004). Nurses' and social workers' attitudes and beliefs about and involvement in life-sustaining treatment decisions. *Health and Social Work, 29,* 27–35.

Werth, J. L. (1999). The role of the mental health professional in helping significant others of persons who are assisted in death. *Death Studies, 23*(3), 239–255.

Werth, J. L. (2002). Legal and ethical considerations for mental health professionals related to end-of-life care and decision making. *American Behavioral Scientist, 46,* 373–383.

Werth, J. L., & Blevins, D. (2002). Public policy and end-of-life care. *American Behavioral Scientist, 46,* 401–417.

Werth, J. L., Blevins, D., Toussaint, K. L., & Durham, M. R. (2002). The influence of cultural diversity on end-of-life care and decisions. *American Behavioral Scientist, 46,* 204–219.

Wesley, C. A. (1996). Social work and end-of-life decisions: Self-determination and the common good. *Health and Social Work, 21*(2), 115–121.

Wesley, C., Tunney, K., & Duncan, E. (2004). Educational needs of hospice social workers: Spiritual assessment and interventions with diverse populations. *American Journal of Hospital Palliative Care, 21,* 40–46.

Part Six

MSW Syllabi: End-of-Life Care—Comprehensive/ Life-Span Content

18

Social Work Practice in End-of-Life Care

Ellen L. Csikai

COURSE DESCRIPTION

This course is focused on social work practice with those who are dying and those who are bereaved by death. It is designed as an elective course to prepare social work students and students in other human service disciplines to work with dying people and their family members and friends who survive them.

OBJECTIVES

After completion of this course, students will be able to:

- Discuss their attitudes and feelings about death and its place in the human life cycle
- Recognize and deal with the needs and concerns of the dying and understand special issues of death, dying, and bereavement as they relate to members of minority groups, people living with AIDS, and children
- Describe and analyze the legal, medical, and moral issues surrounding death
- Help parents with the effects of death in children's lives
- Describe the way death is handled by the health-care system
- Provide direct services to the dying and their families
- Make appropriate referrals to facilities that can be of help to the dying and the bereaved
- Assist patients, the bereaved, and health-care personnel in dealing with their experiences with death
- Distinguish between normal and abnormal grief and work with those for whom grief is a problem

- Analyze contemporary societal practices surrounding death and the meaning this has for the social worker in practice

REQUIRED TEXTS

Albom, M. (1997). *Tuesdays with Morrie*. New York: Bantam Doubleday Dell.

Berzoff, J., & Silverman, P. (2004). *Living with dying: A handbook for end-of-life healthcare practitioners*. New York: Columbia University Press.

Csikai, E., & Chaitin, E. (2005). *Ethics in end-of-decisions for social work practice*. Chicago: Lyceum Books, Inc.

TEACHING METHODS

The class will use a variety of teaching methods, including lecture, discussion, films, student presentations, guest speakers, and in-class exercises. A seminar format will be utilized in which students will be expected to contribute to discussions in a thoughtful, meaningful, and respectful manner. As some students may express very personal feelings and may share their experiences with death and dying, students are expected to be sensitive to this and to maintain confidentiality of such feelings and experiences that are shared in the classroom.

COURSE CONTENT

1. The meaning of death to life: An examination of current attitudes toward death in America
   a. Of what do we die, and when?
   b. Traditional and modern views of death in America
   c. The meaning of death in human development
   d. The factors that shape attitudes toward death
   e. Major religious orientations to death and dying
2. Death in children's lives
   a. How children think of death
   b. How children cope with death
   c. Working with surviving children
   d. Working with parents whose children are dying or have died
3. Death and the health-care system
   a. Attitudes of health-care professionals toward the dying
   b. Problems in health care for the dying: Stigmatization of the dying, managing the cost, etc.
   c. Using hospice and appropriate support groups
   d. Working with dying patients, their families, and the health-care profession
   e. Ethical issues in the care of the dying: Should people be disconnected from life support? When? Who decides? Should people be told they are dying?

4. Legal aspects of death and the social worker's role
   a. The definition of death
   b. The living will: Do people have a right to die?
   c. The ethics of transplants
   d. Official procedures at the time of death
   e. The last will and testament
5. Funerals and body disposition
   a. Some historical background
   b. Funeral practices in America
   c. Methods of body disposition
   d. How the social worker can be of help to the family
6. Working with grief
   a. The nature of bereavement
   b. Normal and abnormal grief
   c. Grief among professionals
   e. Grief and guilt
7. Some special problems in death and dying
   a. Minorities and death
   b. Special problems of widowhood
   c. The AIDS patient and family members
   d. Other problems identified by the class

COURSE OUTLINE

Session 1 Introduction to course
Where we die / Myths about death and dying

Session 2 Social work values / Role in end-of-life care
NASW Practice Standards
Self-care / Secondary trauma
Required reading: Bern-Klug, Gessert, & Forbes; Dane & Chachkes

Session 3 Cultural awareness
Attitudes toward death
Issues of special populations
Required reading: Berzoff & Silverman, chapters 22 and 23; Braun & Nichols

Session 4 Definition of death
Physical signs and symptoms of dying
Required reading: Berzoff & Silverman, chapter 14

Sessions 5 Assessment
Psychological concerns
Teamwork
Required reading: Berzoff & Silverman, chapters 8, 18, and 28; Puchalski & Romer

Session 6 Palliative care
Pain/symptom management
Interventions
Required reading: Berzoff & Silverman, chapters 19 and 20; Choi & Billings

Session 7 Paper due: *Tuesdays with Morrie*
Hospice care (home, inpatient, nursing home)
Required reading: Csikai (2004); Kovacs; Miller & Mor; Raymer & Reese; Reese (1999); Reese et al.

Session 8 Panel from Compassionate Friends
Bereavement
Self-help and mutual aid groups
Grief/depression
Bereavement
Required reading: Berzoff & Silverman, chapters 12 and 29; Li; Walsh-Burke; Wink & Scott

Session 9 Funeral planning: Visit to funeral home
Required reading: Bern-Klug, Eckert, & Wilkinson

Session 10 Grief/depression
Bereavement (cont'd)
Spirituality
Required reading: Berzoff & Silvermanm, chapter 10; Derrickson; Reese (2000)

Session 11 Guest speakers
Bereavement groups
Children and death
Required reading: Berzoff & Silverman, chapter 16; MacGowan; Miller, Hedlund, & Murphy

Session 12 Bioethics
Advance care planning
End-of-life decision making
Student presentations
Required reading: Foster & McLellan; SUPPORT Investigators; Resnick, Cowart, & Kubrin

Session 13 Advance care planning (cont'd)
End-of-life decision making (cont'd)
Student presentations (cont'd)
Required reading: Berzoff & Silverman, chapter 30

Session 14 Suicide
Euthanasia
Assisted suicide
Student presentations (cont'd)
Required reading: Berzoff & Silverman, chapter 38; Csikai (1999b); Miller; Miller, Mesler, & Eggman

Session 15 Final paper due
Self-care
Leadership
Course evaluation
Required reading: Berzoff & Silverman, chapters 43 and 44

BIBLIOGRAPHY

Bern-Klug, M., Eckerdt, D. J., & Wilkinson, D. S. (1999). What families know about funeral-related costs: Implications for social work practice. *Health and Social Work, 24*(2), 128–137.

Bern-Klug, M., Gessert, C., & Forbes, S. (2001). The need to revise assumptions about the end of life: Implications for social work practice. *Health and Social Work, 26*(1), 38–47.

Braun, K. L., & Nichols, R. (1997). Death and dying in four Asian American cultures: A descriptive study. *Death Studies, 21*(4), 327–360.

Choi, Y. S., & Billings, J. A. (2002). Changing perspectives on palliative care. *Oncology, 16*(4), 515–523.

Csikai, E. L. (1999a). Euthanasia and assisted suicide: Issues for social work practice. *Journal of Gerontological Social Work, 31*(3/4), 49–63.

Csikai, E. L. (1999b). The role of values and experience in determining attitudes toward euthanasia and assisted suicide. *Social Work in Health Care, 30*(1), 75–95.

Csikai, E. L. (2004). Social workers' participation in the resolution of ethical dilemmas in hospice care. *Health and Social Work, 29*(1), 67–76.

Dane, B., & Chachkes, E. (2001). The cost of caring for patients with an illness: Contagion to the social worker. *Social Work in Health Care, 33*(2), 31–51.

Derrickson, B. S. (1996). The spiritual work of the dying: A framework and case studies. *Hospice Journal, 11*(2), 11–30.

Foster, L. W., & McLellan, L. J. (2002). Translating psychosocial insight into ethical discussions supportive of families in end-of-life decision-making. *Social Work in Health Care, 35*(3), 37–51.

Kovacs, P. J. (2000). Participatory action research and hospice: A good fit. *Hospice Journal, 15*(3), 55–62.

Li, L. W. (2005). From caregiving to bereavement: Trajectories of depressive symptoms among wife and daughter caregivers. *Journal of Gerontology: Psychological Sciences, 60B*(4), 190–198.

Macgowan, M. J. (2004). Psychosocial treatment of youth suicide: A systematic review of the research. *Research on Social Work Practice, 14*(3), 147–162.

Miller, P. J. (2000). Life after death with dignity: The Oregon experience. *Social Work, 45*(3), 263–271.

Miller, P. J., Hedlund, S., & Murphy, K. (1998). Social work assessment at the end of life: Practice guidelines for suicide and the terminally ill. *Social Work in Health Care, 26*(4), 23–26.

Miller, P. J., Mesler, M. A., & Eggman, S. T. (2002). Take some time to look inside their hearts: Hospice social workers contemplate physician assisted suicide. *Social Work in Health Care, 35*(3), 53–63.

Miller, S. C., & Mor, V. N. T. (2002). The role of hospice care in the nursing home setting. *Journal of Palliative Medicine, 5*(2), 271–274.

Puchalski, C., & Romer, A. L. (2000). Taking a spiritual history allows clinicians to understand patients more fully. *Journal of Palliative Medicine, 3*(1), 129–137.

Raymer, M., & Reese, J. D. (2004). Relationships between social work involvement and hospice outcomes: Results of the national hospice social work survey. *Social Work, 49*(3), 415–422.

Reese, D. J. (1999). Spirituality conceptualized as purpose in life and sense of connection: Major issues and counseling approaches with terminal illness. *Healing Ministry, 6*(3), 101–108.

Reese, D. J. (2000). The role of primary caregiver denial in inpatient placement during home hospice care. *Hospice Journal, 15*(1), 15–33.

Reese, D. J., Ahern, R. E., Nair, S., O'Faire, J. D., & Warren, C. (1999). Hospice access and use by African Americans: Addressing cultural and institutional barriers through participatory action research. *Social Work, 44*(6), 549–560.

Resnick, L., Cowart, M. E., & Kubrin, A. (1998). Perceptions of do-not-resuscitate orders. *Social Work in Health Care, 26*(4), 1–21.

SUPPORT Investigators (1997). Advance directives for seriously ill hospitalized patients: Effectiveness with the Patient Self-Determination Act and the SUPPORT intervention. *Journal of the American Geriatrics Society, 45,* 500–507.

Walsh-Burke, K. (2000). Matching bereavement services to level of need. *Hospice Journal, 15*(1), 77–86.

Wink, P., & Scott, J. (2005). Does religiousness buffer against the fear of death and dying in late adulthood? Findings from a longitudinal study. *Journal of Gerontology: Psychological Sciences, 60B*(4), 207–214.

ASSIGNMENT #1: CRITICAL ANALYSIS PAPER ON TUESDAYS WITH MORRIE

Students will read *Tuesdays with Morrie* by Mitch Albom. A critical analysis of key themes that emerge in the book is to be completed. The paper should be four to five pages in length and written according to APA style. (Students may not substitute viewing the movie for this assignment but may wish to supplement their learning with the movie.)

Using critical thinking, students should identify four key relationships that evolve and the impact of each on Morrie's life and dying as well as five messages that emerge about life, dying, and death throughout the book. Students should describe each concept, how it emerged and related to Morrie and Mitch's relationship, and the impact it had on Mitch's and Morrie's lives.

ASSIGNMENT #2: CULTURAL/BELIEF SYSTEM PRESENTATION

For this assignment, students will work in pairs. Students are required to choose a culture or belief system (religious, spiritual) that is different from their own and prepare an analysis of this culture or belief system in which they discuss death as it is viewed from that belief system. An oral presentation will be made to the class. Students will also hand in an outline (with references) of their presentation to the instructor.

The paper should address

- What is known (from the literature) about attitudes toward dying and death (at least five references)
- What the beliefs about autonomy or self-determination regarding treatment or end-of-life decision making are (i.e., in the belief system, how much information does the dying person want, and who makes treatment decisions)
- What the death rituals are (i.e., burial, cremation)
- How bereavement plays out—are there any expected practices after someone has died?
- If there are any interventions that have been shown to be effective with individuals of this culture or belief system. Describe these. If there is no data on this, what interventions do you believe would be likely to be effective, and why?

ASSIGNMENT #3: SOCIAL WORKER INTERVIEW

This assignment is designed to expose students to social workers working with life-threatening illness, death, dying, grief, and bereavement. Students are to select an area of interest and interview a social worker in that setting. This will allow them to gain an understanding of what the social worker does on a daily basis. Students must also observe the social worker in action.

Part 1: Students must construct an interview that covers the following questions:

1. What is the social worker's background (degrees, how long in social work and in this field, how long at current facility)?
2. What department does the social worker belong to?

3. How does the social worker receive supervision/consultation?
4. What types of patients/families are served at the facility? What types of patients does the social worker spend most of his or her time with?
5. What services does the social worker provide? What are the main interventions used by the social worker (i.e., crisis intervention, case management, bereavement interventions)?
6. What are some of the patient-related challenges faced by the social worker?
7. What are some of the institutional-related challenges faced by the social worker?
8. What are some of the ethical challenges faced by the social worker?
9. What are some of the barriers to providing effective services faced by the social worker?
10. Are there any cultural barriers within the facility?
11. What specific knowledge is needed by social workers in this setting?
12. Who are the health-care professionals with whom he or she interacts most? What interdisciplinary teams are present for case review/consultation?
13. What does the social worker enjoy the most about his or her job?

Students will write a narrative of four to five pages summarizing their interview. The narrative must include

1. A description of the health-care setting, including the name of the agency/facility, its location (i.e., rural/urban), the type of facility, and populations it serves (number and types). Students may want to introduce the paper with this. Students need to specifically address whether it is rural or urban and if rural clients are also served if it is in an urban area.
2. Impressions of the interview—how receptive was the social worker to examining his or her job? Were there any realizations made by the social worker (i.e., did the social worker realize he or she really does a lot more for the patients than he or she thought or discover areas that need action within the facility)?

Part 2: Students are to observe one social worker–client interaction with the social worker you interviewed. The interaction may take place in the facility or in the home (wherever the social worker typically provides services). Students will likely need to attain permission from the facility and consent from the patient/family prior to completion of this part of the assignment. Permission for this part of the assignment must be granted when the student initially discusses the assignment with the social worker. If it is not possible to do the observation, then students will need to choose another social worker and facility. (If students are able to review the case file/record, they should do so.) Students will submit a narrative describing their observation/experience. The narrative should be four to five pages long and should answer the following questions.

1. First describe the presenting problem of the patient/family and the psychosocial history. (This should be brief—no more than one page.) Was there a caregiver or family member also present?
2. Describe how the social worker engaged the patient. In what setting did this take place (home, hospital room, etc.)?
3. How did the patient receive the social worker? If this was a new patient, what was his or her reaction to being approached by a social worker?
4. What was the social worker's assessment of the patient situation? What assessment tools were used? If formal tools were used, include them if this is possible.
5. What were the plan and time frame for the intervention?
6. How did the social worker plan to evaluate the effectiveness of service with this patient? And overall? Will there be any follow-up?
7. Describe any potential ethical issues that may arise in the patient's situation.
8. Are there any cultural considerations? What are they?
9. Were there any foreseeable challenges/barriers in meeting this patient's needs?
10. Describe the organization and contents of the case file/record. (Indicate if you were not able to review this.)
11. Describe the documentation that the social worker completed for the interaction.
12. Were you able to see the social worker in a different light when he or she was interacting with the client/patient?
13. Describe the level of ease with which the social worker utilized the helping process.
14. Do you think the social worker enjoys his or her work? Explain your response.
15. What would you have done differently?

Students also must include a one-page summary of the interview and observation that answers the following questions:

1. Do you have a different opinion of this type of setting/position now as opposed to before your interview and observation? Explain.

2. To what degree do you believe that social work is valued in this agency/facility? What could be done to change this in any way?
3. Is this a setting in which you would like to be employed?

Students are encouraged to add other information that they found interesting or that they think is important.

Social Worker Interview Consent

The interview you are being asked to participate in is an assignment for a course called Social Work Practice with the Dying and Bereaved. The purpose of the interview is for me to understand in depth, from your perspective, what your job as a social worker in a health-care setting it is like for you. You will be asked, for example, to talk about your responsibilities, challenges you face, and interactions with other professionals. The goal is that this interview will give me a better picture of what being a social worker in a health-care setting is like as I make future job choices. Your thoughtful responses throughout the interview are valuable and will be respected.

The interview should last about thirty to forty-five minutes. You should understand that your name will not be associated with your responses. You should understand that I will use the information you provide for a written assignment for the course. My professor will be the only person to read this, although I may also be asked to discuss in general my interview with you in the class session with other students. Again, your name will not be used.

If at any time during or after this interview you have any questions about the interview or feel uneasy about your participation, you may contact me, ____________________, at ____________________ or my professor, ____________________, at ____________________. Your participation in this interview is completely voluntary and you may withdraw your consent to participate in the interview at any time during or after the completion of the interview by contacting me or my professor.

Thank you for your time.

Informed Consent:

I understand the purpose of this interview and the use that will be made of the information I provide. I understand that my name will in no way be associated with my responses. In granting my consent, I understand that my participation in this interview is voluntary and that I may withdraw from it at any time without penalty.

____________________ ____________________

Signature Date

____________________ ____________________

Witness Date

CASE STUDY ASSIGNMENT

The purpose of this assignment is for students to demonstrate an understanding of the helping process regarding problems or issues faced by individuals who are dying, who are caring for those who are dying, or who have experienced the death of someone close to them for which social work intervention is needed. This will involve the application of course content to a specific case.

Attached to these instructions are several case scenarios that describe health-care problems with patients in specific health-care settings. You will choose one case and respond to the questions below. You should respond as if you are the social worker in the case. Please keep in mind that since there is limited information given for each case scenario, in order to be able to work through the assignment, you will need to provide additional hypothetical information, including interventions, outcomes/disposition, and follow-up with the case.

If you utilize any Web, journal, or book resources, please cite them appropriately in APA style in the body of the paper and include a separate page with the heading "References." If you incorporate readings but do not use them directly in the paper, the correct heading to use is "Bibliography." You do not need to cite the case study or class lecture, but if you use sources such as the textbook, you will need citations. I anticipate that the length of your paper will be about ten to twelve pages. (This does not include your reference list.)

Areas to be addressed:

Engagement:

What is the presenting problem?

Where do the initial interviews/meetings take place?

Who is present?

What is the condition of the patient? Is the patient able to participate? (if appropriate to the case)

Data collection:

What is the initial information provided to you? What are the sources?

What additional information is needed (from family, medical team, etc.)?

What is the purpose of this additional information?

What are factors (patient, family, institutional, cultural, and personal values) that may affect your interaction with the patient? With the family? With the health-care team?

Assessment and Planning:

What are the important aspects of the case?

Where can social work intervene to resolve the client's issues and increase the patient's quality of life?

Describe what you have contracted with the patient as the work to be done (formal or informal contracts with patient and family).

List two goals with corresponding objectives and tasks (and who will do what).

Describe the process of how goals were formulated. Who will do what?

Intervention:

Based on the goals listed, what intervention is needed? And why did you decide this was the best intervention to use?

Keep in mind that different interventions may need to be used in order to achieve each goal. (This is where you will need to provide sources regarding the effectiveness of the intervention with this patient population or regarding typical interventions or services provided in that health-care setting. At least one reference should be cited.) Choose from the following interventions: case management, information and referral, education, discharge planning, supporting counseling, family counseling, advocacy, resource development, outreach, family conferencing, loss histories, bereavement counseling, anticipatory grief counseling, support groups, legacy building, cognitive-behavioral intervention.

Describe the implementation of the intervention plan.

How did it proceed? (This will require a detailed description of your interviews/meetings with patient, family, and health-care team members—at least two pages.)

Evaluation:

How will you know if your intervention is successful?

Discuss and provide an example of at least one measure used to evaluate your intervention in the case.

Was your intervention successful?

What are the potential outcomes in the case if the patient and/or family completes tasks assigned and complies with plan or if the client does not comply or is not cooperative with the plan?

What are potential problems/obstacles to meeting the needs of the patient and family?

Termination:

What are the termination issues to consider in the case? (Is it planned or unplanned?)

Discuss two of these issues and how you would handle them in the case.

What are the termination issues to consider with respect to the team and patient?

Describe how you would assist with team issues around termination.

Follow-up:

Describe the follow-up for the case. What is done, and how often?

Summary:

What are the knowledge and unique skills that the social worker can bring to this case?

What do you believe are two barriers to the social worker's ability to provide effective services in this case?

What stressors does the social worker face in this case? In this setting?

Identify at least one specific source of frustration you think you would have in dealing with this client population in this setting.

Choose one of the following cases to complete this assignment:

Case #1: Ian is forty-two. After twelve years of living with HIV, he is now dying of AIDS. His partner of fifteen years, Gus, is also HIV positive. Gus has an eighteen-year-old son, Mark, who has lived with Gus and Ian since he was three. Earlier in the year, Ian had pneumonia, and everyone thought he was dying. Now, Ian is completely bed bound and sleeps much of the time. He has ongoing difficulty breathing and frequent incontinence. Despite Gus's devoted care, bedsores have begun to develop on Ian's heels and tailbone. Movement and changes in position cause Ian some pain.

Ian has had several restless nights. During these times, he pulls at his clothes and tries to get out of the bed. Once, he fell, hitting his head on a table. If Gus tries to hold Ian's hands, Ian yells, "Don't hurt me." This is very upsetting to Gus and Mark. Ian has been mumbling intermittently about a report or project that he must finish. This is very confusing to Gus because Ian hasn't been well enough to work for two years. Ian has also talked about going to a cabin that his family owned when he was a child.

Several years ago, Gus and Ian invited a dying friend to live with them. Gus has horrible memories of that friend's death. He remembers his friend being blue and gasping for air when he died. Exhausted and afraid of reliving that experience, Gus would like to admit Ian to an inpatient hospice to die, although Ian earlier expressed his wish to remain at home.

Even though Gus knows Ian didn't want to see his family, Gus often wonders if he should call and let them know what is happening. Gus feels ambivalent about some of the choices he has made, but he didn't know what else to do. He doesn't want to burden Mark with these questions, and although he knows that Ian would understand why he has made these decisions, he wishes that they could talk about these things one more time.

Case #2: Bob and Margaret grew up together and have been married for thirty-eight years. Bob is a mail carrier, and Margaret is a graphic designer. They have one adult child and three young grandchildren who live nearby. Margaret, now sixty-four years old, was diagnosed with breast cancer five years ago. At that time, she had surgery and extensive treatment. The cancer recurred three years ago but did not respond well to chemotherapy. Recent tests have shown, unfortunately, that the cancer has now spread to her bones, liver, and brain. The oncologist has explained to Margaret and Bob that she has one to two months to live. Margaret has declined any further treatment.

Most of the time, Margaret is in bed. When she is awake, she is nauseated and uncomfortable. She does not want to increase her pain medications, however, because they make her drowsy. Bob is troubled by her significant weight loss and constantly tries to entice her with her favorite foods. She has no appetite, though, and is taking in only sips of lemonade, water, and melted popsicles. Margaret occasionally talks openly about dying, but only with friends.

Margaret knows that Bob is not sleeping or eating properly and feels like she has let him down. At the same time, she also says that he is a stubborn person and that she is too tired to convince him to allow their friends and family to help out. Bob finds displays of emotion very embarrassing and unsettling and asks people not to say or ask anything that will make him cry. He says that after Margaret dies, he will have all the time and privacy he needs to grieve, but for now his focus is on her needs. He is determined to learn the right way to do everything and puts a lot of pressure on himself to do it all. He has a hard time asking for and accepting help, although many friends and family have offered. He believes that every moment he spends with Margaret may be her last and doesn't want her to feel alone or abandoned. He worries when he is away from her and is not interested in spending time with other people or engaging in activities.

Although she acknowledges that death will occur at some point, Margaret hopes to feel better soon. She feels sad about leaving her grandchildren and about not being there to see them grow up. She does not want them to be told she is dying and is uncomfortable with them seeing her in her present condition. Bob feels she is distancing herself from the children and struggles with how to explain this to them.

Case #3: John is a sixty-two-year-old man who was self-referred to you through the company's employee assistance program. He has been unable to sleep and has little interest in his usual activities, such as the local Rotary club, fishing, and attending football games at the local university (of which he is an alumnus). He also uses alcohol on a daily basis, especially when he has trouble sleeping. He works as a regional manager for corporate loan accounts at Union Bank. Recently the bank was bought out, and while he kept his job, he has much less responsibility than he did before. He and his wife had one son, James, with whom he remained involved after their divorce when James was thirteen years old. James had difficulty accepting the divorce and began using drugs in high school. James committed suicide when he was twenty-two years old (ten years ago). John has never really dealt with James's death.

Case #4: Betty is a seventy-five-year-old woman who has been diagnosed with stomach cancer with metastases to the bone. So far she is still ambulatory and able to do normal daily activities such as grocery shopping with her husband and going out for lunch, although it tires her out. Betty and her husband, Sam (seventy-eight years old), have been married for fifty-five years. They have two children—one son and one daughter—and five grandchildren. Both children live close by. Betty worked in an accounting firm and Sam worked at a steel mill before they both retired. Sam is very anxious about Betty's impending death and can't imagine how he will manage without her, He doesn't totally acknowledge it since she is still able to do pretty much for herself. Betty explains to you that she is concerned because she has taken care of all the financial matters during the marriage and Sam won't listen to her when she tries to teach him how to manage the bills and show him important documents, such as insurance, and when she tries to talk to him about funeral planning.

19

Death, Dying, and Bereavement

Social Work/Clergy Collaboration to Improve End-of-Life Care

John Linder

COURSE DESCRIPTION

The purpose of this course is twofold. First, participants are invited to explore the meaning of mortality and spirituality for themselves. Students are asked to view these topics through the lenses of both their personal and professional lives. Second, students will be guided through a didactic and experiential exploration of critical end-of-life issues and clinical interventions. We will examine mortality; spirituality; today's health-care system; the interdisciplinary care delivery model; and the roles of social workers, spiritual care providers, and faith communities in helping the dying.

Patients with life-threatening diseases or injuries and the people they value are usually deeply affected by the diagnosis, treatment, and changing condition of the patient. These changes often stimulate both heightened psychosocial needs and increased spiritual or existential distress. In fact, five domains of the patient-caregiver ecosystem are usually affected by the dying process: the physical, psychological, spiritual/existential, material, and relational.

Dying and death experiences vary greatly from one person to the next. Some of these variations are based in culture or ethnicity. In addition to more obvious racial/ethnic and global cultural considerations, issues such as primary language; immigration status; sexual orientation; culturally derived styles of communication and support; intergenerational differences in acculturation or assimilation; biculturalism; and the variety of viewpoints concerning illness, disease, dying, death, and bereavement contribute to this variation and will be examined. Individual beliefs and faith history, current faith community participation, and spiritual expression are another crucial area of diversity.

Other differences are based in demography and ecology: gender, age, disease type, physical location (of both person and disease), socioeconomic standing, and level of education. Still other variation is rooted in the psychological development of the individual and the support system surrounding him or her. Belief systems, including religious practice, spiritual beliefs, and existential worldviews, may also account for substantial variation. Most often, a complex blend of many of these factors shapes the dying experience for the individual and his or her loved ones and caregivers. Developing and maintaining sensitivity to these variations is a critical skill for social workers and pastoral care providers encountering dying individuals and populations.

The preferred treatment modality for providing end-of-life care to the terminally ill involves an interdisciplinary team. Social work and chaplaincy are two of the disciplines integral to this team. This course is intended to deepen all participants' knowledge of terminal illness, processes for accessing health care and making health-care decisions, advance medical planning, the dying process as part of the life cycle, and the dynamic relationship among the patient, caregivers, and professional care team. The participants will explore patients' psychosocial and spiritual strengths and needs. These strengths and needs intersect and overlap, touching both the social work and spiritual care professions. Participants will examine the benefits and barriers of social work–faith leader cooperation in enhancing the end-of-life experience for patients and loved ones/caregivers alike.

COURSE OBJECTIVES

In this course,

- Students will engage in exercises intended to produce an examination of individual mortality as well as personal belief systems concerning spiritual or existential viewpoints.
- Students will demonstrate an understanding of the dying process, particularly as it relates to chronic or terminal illness. This understanding will encompass patient and caregiver/loved ones' perspectives in the appropriate sociocultural ecosystem. Included in this understanding will be an awareness of how ethnicity, culture, religious preference and denomination, age, gender, and other factors affect perspective and may affect medical decision making.
- Students will develop an informed understanding of the spiritual or existential issues raised by many patients and family members (family as defined by the client/patient) in response to progressive, chronic, or terminal illness. This understanding will enhance students' abilities to differentiate between psychosocial and spiritual concerns.
- Students will experience and reflect on one spiritual or faith tradition with which they are not familiar. (Accommodation will be made

should an individual's beliefs prohibit participation in or observation of faith practices other than his or her own—please see instructor.)

- Students will discuss the implications of belief systems and of progressive or terminal illness in guiding treatment and interaction with patients/clients and families. Based on each student's prior training and experience, students will incorporate therapeutic or pastoral counseling theory and practice and enhance clinical or pastoral skills.
- Students will demonstrate a basic understanding of the central ethical issues associated with the treatment of chronic, progressive, and terminal illness.
- Students will develop and articulate strategies to enhance participation of and collaboration between faith leaders and social workers in the care of the dying and their loved ones
- Students will be able to conduct a comprehensive psychosocial assessment of a patient-caregiver system, identify concurrent spiritual or existential issues, identify and prioritize needs, and develop a plan of care

TEACHING METHOD

The instructor uses dynamic and diverse teaching methods, in recognition that adult learners benefit most from a multi-modality learning environment. The course format will integrate individual and group experiential exercises; dyad, small group, and whole class discussion and didactic modules; and panel presentations and discussions, as well as various audiovisual and written media. Content and process have equal importance in this course, making attendance and participation imperative. The instructor will pay particular attention to diversity content in all aspects, and case discussions will affirm this diversity. Students will be encouraged to share professional and/or personal experiences that will further enrich the diversity dialogue.

COURSE REQUIREMENTS

Two brief written exercises, one completed in class and one at home

Three tasks with accompanying reflection papers. The reflection paper should be no more than three pages, double spaced. The main goal is to enter fully into the task then examine attitudes, feelings, and thoughts you have about the task; how these affect your understanding of issues surrounding spirituality, dying, and death; and how this understanding is related to the professional practices and interventions of clinical social work and pastoral spiritual care.

Task #1: Visit a social service agency or placement that deals with death and dying. Interview a staff member and find out how psychosocial and spiritual needs are assessed and met, what disciplines are involved in care, and the extent to which families or caregivers are involved in care and care planning. Many environments are appropriate for this task. Some of the most obvious are hospitals, skilled nursing and assisted living centers, home care providers, and hospice agencies. However, many agencies provide services to the dying or their caregivers. Homeless shelters, Meals-on-Wheels programs, adult day care, dialysis centers, Alzheimer's care centers, long-term mental health treatment facilities (locked and open), and board-and-care homes all deal with populations that occasionally or chronically include the dying. Use your imagination.

In today's busy service environment, you may find yourself conducting this interview over the phone; providers may be willing to give you fifteen minutes on the phone but may not have the time or inclination to meet face to face. The preference is for face-to-face contact, which will allow you observation of the environment. If that is not possible, a phone interview will suffice.

Please indicate the agency name, location, and target population at the start of your paper. This description should not take more than a paragraph or two. Your reflection (excluding the description of the agency) should be no more than three pages, double spaced.

Task #2: Complete an advance directive. Use either one of the forms valid in your state or the Five Wishes document. Write an accompanying reflection. Examples of two forms will be provided (including the Five Wishes document); if you have another that you prefer and that is valid in your state, feel free to use it. In your reflection, pay particular attention to the choices you make regarding your care and regarding the person or people you designate to carry out that care if you cannot. The emotions generated by this exercise hold equal weight with the content of the exercise itself; please discuss these in your reflection. If you already have an advance medical directive, please review it, consider whether or not you want to revise it, and reflect on the process you went through in completing it as well as any process changes you would make in completing one today. In addition to the completed forms (photocopies are fine), your reflection should be no more than three pages, double spaced, in length.

Task #3: Observe and/or participate in a service or ritual, or interview one of the members or ministers, of a spiritual/religious tradition other than your own. Briefly describe the particulars of the service you attend (when, where, what, and with whom, maximum one page), and write the accompanying reflection. This exercise may or may not contain components examining end-of-life issues. This is primarily intended to broaden your exposure to and appreciation of the diversity of beliefs and practices that comprise more organized religious or spiritual expression. If, in this process, you have the opportunity to learn about particular beliefs or practices concerning rituals for or care of the dying, the dead, caregivers, and the bereaved, so much the better. Again, your reflection (excluding the description of the service) should be no more than three pages, double spaced.

Final Assignment. The final assignment is composed of two parts.

In the first part, write a vignette describing an end-of-life scenario. This should be no more than one page double spaced. In the scenario, please describe the patient, his or her caregivers, and other important involved parties; the patient's disease and current health status; and the patient's beliefs about his or her disease and treatment. Please also include a description of the patient's values, spiritual perspective, and membership and participation in any religious denomination, if he or she is affiliated with a faith community. Finally, describe some of the problems the patient, caregivers, or loved ones are encountering.

These scenarios should be generic and can be constructed from personal or professional experience (with care to preserve the confidentiality and shield the identity of real people) or from your imagination. Please present believable scenarios, ones we all might be likely to encounter in working with people facing the end of life. Feel free to construct more-or-less conventional families and caregiver constellations. People's affiliations with faith communities can run the gamut from atheist to nonpracticing to moderately involved to deeply committed and filled with the belief that their community's prayers will bring a cure or healing. Problems can be relational, existential, medical, spiritual, or material; they can be long term and deeply entrenched or transient, disease related or not. Provide enough detail to give an adequate structure for response, but not so elaborate as to confound your colleagues.

The second part of the assignment is for you to use the scenario you are given to discuss this case and your approach to providing care for the patient (and perhaps the caregivers). This may include your assessment and prioritization of needs, some determination on your part as to who would best respond to these needs, and how that help will be mobilized. As a social worker or spiritual care provider, what services could you offer? In your role as a social worker or spiritual care provider, what do you feel would be important in your work with this patient? What strengths does the patient or caregiver have on which you might build? What difficulties can you anticipate? What countertransferential issues arise for you? Would you work with other disciplines, and if so, how? What don't you know that you need to know, and how would you go about discovering or learning it? This part of the assignment should be six to eight pages, double spaced, in length.

DIVERSITY AND VALUES

Diversity material is integrated into each of the weekly topic areas and is specifically addressed in sessions 6 and 7 (diverse cultural and social understandings of death and dying). There is significant material dealing explicitly with diversity, justice, and ethics in sessions 2 and 3 (social construction and coping with death), 8 (ethics and end-of-life decision making), 9 (issues of children and death), and 14 and 15 (grief, ritual, and bereavement). The Fadiman text and many of the readings address specific issues of diversity and specific populations at risk. Furthermore, extensive attention is paid to the variety of axes on which issues of diversity and justice exist. Throughout the course, diverse content is explicitly encouraged as part of in-class discussion as well as exercises and written assignments.

REQUIRED TEXTS

Albom, M. (1997). *Tuesdays with Morrie: An old man, a young man, and life's greatest lesson*. New York: Doubleday.

DeSpelder, L., & Strickland, A. L. (Eds.). (1995). *The path ahead*. Mountain View, CA: Mayfield.

Fadiman, A. (1998). *The spirit catches you and you fall down*. New York: Farrar, Straus and Giroux.

Worden, J. W. (2002). *Grief counseling and grief therapy: A handbook for the mental health practitioner* (3rd ed). New York: Springer.

COURSE OUTLINE

Session 1 Introduction / touching mortality

Required reading for next week:

DeSpelder & Strickland, pp. 1–6 (introduction), 7–18 (Kastenbaum), 19–28 (Feifel), 303–311 (Corr)

DeVries, R. G. (1981). Birth and death: Social construction at the poles of existence. *Social Forces, 59*(4), 1074–1093.

Assignment: Complete student information and background form

Session 2 The social construction of death

Required reading for next week:

DeSpelder & Strickland, pp. 116–124 (Lammers), 295–300 (Brodkey)

Corr, C. (1993). Coping with dying: Lessons that we should and should not learn from the work of Elisabeth Kubler-Ross. *Death Studies, 17,* 69–83.

Littlewood, J. (1993). The denial of death and rites of passage in contemporary societies. In D. Clark (Ed.), *The sociology of death: Theory, culture, practice* (pp. 69–84). Cambridge, MA: Blackwell.

Singer, P. A., Martin, D. K., & Kelner, M. (1999). Quality end-of-life care: Patients' perspectives. *Journal of the American Medical Association, 281*(2), 163–168.

Due in class: Completed student information and background form

Assignment: Complete spiritual assessment questions

Session 3 Societal coping with death

Required reading for next week:

Albom (Start reading—this is due in two weeks.)

Feldstein, B. D. (2001). Toward meaning. *Journal of the American Medical Association, 286,* 1291–1292.

Hodge, D. (2001). Spiritual assessment: A review of major quantitative methods and a new framework for assessing spirituality. *Social Work, 46*(3), 203–214.

O'Connor, T., McCarroll-Butler, P., Gadowski, S., O'Neill, K., & Meakes, E. Making the most and making sense: Ethnographic research on spirituality in palliative care. *Journal of Pastoral Care, 51*(1), 25–36.

Reese, D. J., & Brown, D. R. (1997). Psychosocial and spiritual care in hospice: Differences between nursing, social work and clergy. *Hospice Journal, 12*(1), 29–41.

Scott, M., Grzbowski, M., & Webb, S. (1994). Perceptions and practices of registered nurses regarding pastoral care and the spiritual needs of hospital patients. *Journal of Pastoral Care, 48*(2), 171–179.

Smith, E. D. (1995). Addressing the psychospiritual distress of death as reality: A transpersonal approach. *Social Work, 40*(3), 402–413.

Due in class: Written spiritual assessment questions and answers

Assignment: Task #1

Session 4 Existential and spiritual assessment

Required reading for next week:

Albom (Finish reading—this is due in class next week.)

DeSpelder & Strickland, pp. 165–168 (Leviton)

Mohrmann, M., Healey, D., & Childress, M. (2000). Suffering's witness: The problem of evil in medical practice. *Second Opinion, 3,* 55–70.

Assignment: Task #1 due in one week

Session 5 Meaning in suffering and death
Required reading for next week:
DeSpelder & Strickland, pp. 41–58 (Scheper-Hughes), 75–79 (Hayes), 80–92 (Barrett)
Fadiman (Start reading—this is due in two weeks.)
Kagawa-Singer, M. (1994). Diverse cultural beliefs and practices about death and dying in the elderly. *Gerontology and Geriatrics Education, 15*(1), 101–116.
Weaver, H. N. (1999). Through indigenous eyes: Native Americans and the HIV epidemic. *Health and Social Work, 24*(1), 27–34.
Young, G. Y. (1997). Shame and guilt mechanisms in East Asian culture. *Journal of Pastoral Care,* 51(1), 57–64.
Due in class: Task #1
Assignment: None

Session 6 Diverse sociocultural understandings of death, part I
Required reading for next week:
Fadiman (Finish reading—this is due in class next week.)
Assignment: None

Session 7 Diverse sociocultural understandings of death, part II
Required reading for next week:
Bowman, K. W. (2000). Communication, negotiation and mediation: Dealing with conflict in end-of-life decisions. *Journal of Palliative Care, 16*(Suppl.), S17–S23.
Galambos, C. M. (1998). Preserving end-of-life autonomy: The Patient Self-Determination Act and the Uniform Health Care Decisions Act. *Health and Social Work, 23*(4), 275–281.
Wesley, C. A. (1996). Social work and end-of-life decisions: Self-determination and the common good. *Health and Social Work, 21*(2), 115–121.
Assignment: Task #2 (This is due in two weeks.)

Session 8 Ethics and end-of-life decision making
Required reading for next week:
DeSpelder & Strickland, pp. 133–143 (Bartholome), 246–259 (Klass), 260–270 (Silverman)
Assignment: Task #2 due next week

Session 9 The problem of dying children, siblings, and parents
Required reading for next week:
Gerkin, C. V. (1997). Final chapters in life stories: The community of faith and the care of older persons. In *An introduction to pastoral care* (pp. 205–225). Nashville, TN: Abingdon Press.

Scheib, K. D. (2000). Older widows: Surviving, thriving and reinventing one's life. In J. Stevenson-Moessner (Ed.), *In her own time: Women and developmental issues in pastoral care* (pp. 251–265). Minneapolis, MN: Fortress Press.
Due in class: Task #2
Assignment: Task #3

Session 10 Religious traditions and end of life
Required reading for next week:
DeSpelder & Strickland, pp. 29–32 (Rosenberg), 154–164 (Dougherty), 182–197 (Stillion), 198–210 (Early)
Somlai, A., Heckman, T., Kelley, J., Mulry, G., Sikkeman, K., & Multhauf, K. (1997). The response of religious congregations to the spiritual needs of people living with HIV/AIDS. *Journal of Pastoral Care, 51*(4), 415–426.
Somlai, A., Kelley, J., Kalichman, S., Mulry, G., Sikkeman, K., McAuliffe, T., et al. (1996). An empirical investigation of the relationship between spirituality, coping, and emotional distress in people living with HIV infection and AIDS. *Journal of Pastoral Care, 50*(2), 181–191.
Van Loon, R. A. (1999). Desire to die in terminally ill people: A framework for assessment and intervention. *Health and Social Work, 24*(4), 260–268.
Due in class: Task #3
Assignment: Work on vignette, which will be due in two weeks.

Session 11 Terminal illness and suicide
Required reading for next week: None
Assignment: Vignette due next week

Session 12 Caregiving and adaptive survivorship
Required reading for next week:
Worden, introduction and chapters 1, 7, and 8
Due in class: Vignette
Assignment: None

Session 13 A good death
Required reading for next week:
Worden, chapters 2–6.
Assignment: Vignettes handed back with feedback

Session 14 Grief, ritual, and bereavement, part I
Required reading for next week:
DeSpelder & Strickland, pp. 271–275 (Doka)
Bastis, M. K. (1996). Thom's garden. *Journal of Pastoral Care, 50*(2), 221–222.

Smith, D. (1997). The litany of release. *Journal of Pastoral Care, 51*(4), 431–434.

Assignment: Vignettes are distributed. Reaction/reflection papers will be due in two weeks.

Session 15 Grief, ritual, and bereavement, part II
Required reading for next week: None
Assignment: None

Session 16 Summary
Due in class: Vignettes and response

20

Caring for Persons with Life-Limiting Illness

A Life-Span Approach

Taryn Lindhorst and Bonnie Letinich

COURSE DESCRIPTION

Caring for Persons with Life-Limiting Illness: A Life-Span Approach is a foundation practice course with a focus on multisystemic social work practice with seriously ill people who have a life-limiting condition. In childhood, conditions that could end in death include diseases such as cancer, cystic fibrosis, and AIDS, as well as congenital birth anomalies and neurodegenerative disorders. For adults, common end-of-life conditions are end-stage organ diseases, various cancers, and end-stage AIDS. Traumatic injuries can also create situations where the anticipation of death requires symptom control and care planning.

A strengths-based, multigenerational, and multicultural framework undergirds this practice course. We will examine how families care for a member who is critically ill, and the differences that occur when the seriously ill person is a child or adolescent, a middle-aged adult, or an elder at the end of life. The culture of each family in terms of its ethnic and spiritual heritage, values, and beliefs drives decision making about end-of-life care. Families have differential levels of access to institutional and community resources based on economics, legacies of racism and homophobia, and gendered caregiving demands. These differing experiences have profound implications for end-of-life care.

Families state that they want helpful communication and coordinated care throughout the course of an illness, regardless of its length, in an institution that feels safe. To accomplish this goal, this course focuses on developing skills in empowerment-oriented social work practice within the context of the current service delivery system. To work effectively, social workers need skills in identifying multigenerational family strengths based in an appreciation of the client's culture, as well as the capacity to work effectively within interdisciplinary teams of care providers. This framework is consistent with the social change and social justice mission of the MSW curriculum.

This course will develop skills in three areas: theoretical knowledge; development of self-awareness in issues related to death, dying, and grief; and application of this knowledge to social work practice with families. Foundational theories related to grief, loss, and attachment are used to interpret case examples from a variety of settings. Students will become familiar with tools for psychosocial-spiritual assessment and decision making. Hospice and palliative care models appropriate for social work practice at the end of life will be presented and critiqued.

COURSE OBJECTIVES

At the end of this course, students will have acquired the following skills in self-awareness, theory, and practice:

Self-Awareness Skills

- Students will be able to demonstrate awareness of their own assumptions, beliefs, values, and behaviors with regard to death, dying, and grief and their own mortality.
- Students will be able to affirm and respect their own and others' cultural identities as they interface with choices regarding death and grief.
- Students will be able to be mindful of the role of power differentials and social inequalities influencing family and professional staff behavior and relations in end-of-life care.
- Students will be able to demonstrate awareness of the role of the self in group dynamics and decision-making conferences related to care planning.

Theory Skills

- Students will understand the complexity and reciprocity of multicultural, multigenerational dynamics across different populations and families.
- Students will be able to use theory on grief and loss and information on differing cultural views on death and dying to inform understanding of family functioning.
- Students will be able to apply theories related to grief, loss, and attachment to understand family decision-making processes.
- Students will be able to identify developmental issues for children, middle-aged adults, and elders as they apply to end-of-life care.

- Students will be able to evaluate models of end-of-life care, including hospice and palliative care models and what they offer that differs from the standard practice of hospital-based death.
- Students will be able to identify issues related to the professional caregiver's experience of grief, attachment, and loss.

Practice Skills

- Students will develop the ability to bring a multigenerational, multicultural lens to their assessment of the strengths of individuals and families.
- Students will be able to perform biopsychosocial-spiritual assessments of families encountering life-limiting conditions.
- Students will understand the skills necessary to co-facilitate family decision-making conferences with professional interdisciplinary care teams regarding end-of-life care options.
- Students will be able to evaluate common ethical dilemmas facing social work practitioners working in end-of-life care.
- Students will be able to identify methods to empower families and teams to work collaboratively to develop a plan of care.

TEACHING METHODS

This course will be taught using interactive and participatory exercises and focuses heavily on the development of self-awareness, so students should be prepared to wrestle with their own fears, beliefs, and hopes about the living/dying process. We will use stories, art, films, guided discussion, role play, and other activities to explore the content and processes of the course.

EVALUATION METHODS

The grade for this course is based on five areas, four of which include mini–writing assignments. The assignments are graded based on four criteria: (a) thoroughness and completeness of content, (b) clarity and logic of presentation (c) evidence of critical thought and self-reflection, and (d) writing and editing quality. Feedback on the student's strengths and need for improvement in each of these areas will be provided to each student. These assignments are designed to meet the course goals of increasing self-awareness, understanding of theory, and application of practice skills.

Self-Awareness Skills Development

15% Personal death awareness: This paper is a personal reflection on your own beliefs, values, and concerns regarding issues related to death and dying. The paper should be three to five pages long.

15% Planning your advance directives: During the second week of class, you will receive advanced care planning documents designed to help you determine your wishes for end-of-life care. Your assignment will be to fill out the guidelines for yourself and discuss these with the person you identify as your health-care proxy. You will also visit a funeral home to understand what funeral/cremation arrangements entail. You will turn in a paper that discusses your experiences with this assignment and the implications this has for work with people with serious illnesses. This paper should be two to three pages long.

Application of Theory to Social Work Practice

15% Reflections on the readings: Three times over the course of the class, you will be asked to post to the course discussion board one of the following: (1) a question that has arisen for you from the readings or (2) something from the readings that has affected you or stood out to you in some way. Twice you will be asked to respond to another person's postings on the readings.

15% Class participation: Throughout the class, we will be engaging with the stories of people facing serious illness; therefore, it is very important that you attend every class. Class time will include small group discussion, participation in role plays, and observation of an interview with a person with a serious illness. You will be asked to write three one-page reflection papers on these experiences (sometimes in class, sometimes after class). Participation does not always mean talking but can be reflected in active listening to the comments of others.

40% Case assessment: In this paper, you will present a written case assessment and summary discussion of your learning. More information on this assignment will be presented in class. The case assessment will be based on a case study presented in Barnard, D., Towers, A., Boston, P., & Lambrinidou, Y. (2000). *Crossing over: Narratives of palliative care.* New York: Oxford University Press. The four narratives tell the stories of Joey Court, a child who is ill; Shamira Cook, a parent who is ill; Klara Bergman, an elder experiencing despair; and Paula Ferrari, an adult triumphing over despair.

REQUIRED TEXTS

Kissane, D. W., & Bloch, S. (2003). *Family focused grief therapy.* Philadelphia: Open University Press.

Quill, T. E. (2001). *Caring for patients at the end of life: Facing an uncertain future together.* New York: Oxford University Press.

SUPPLEMENTAL TEXTS

Berzoff, J., & Silverman, P. (Eds.). (2005). *Living with dying: A handbook for end-of-life healthcare practitioners*. New York: Columbia University Press.

Hilden, J., & Robin, D. R., with Lindsey, K. (2003). *Shelter from the storm: Caring for a child with a life-threatening condition*. Cambridge, MA: Perseus Press.

Lynn, J., & Harrold, J. (1999). *Handbook for mortals: Guidance for people facing serious illness*. New York: Oxford University Press.

COURSE OUTLINE

The Big Picture: Understanding the Intersections between Systems of Care and the Culture of the Family

Session 1 Systems of care: The care for dignity-conserving care

Objective: To contrast varying models of care for individuals with life-threatening illness from a social justice stance

Reading:

Quill, chapters 1, 2, 3, 4, 10

Frank Ostaseski's "Five Precepts"

Chochinov, H. M. (2002). Dignity and psychotherapeutic considerations in end-of-life care. *Journal of Palliative Care, 20,* 134–142.

Session 2 Culture, values, and illness

Objective: To use readings related to class, ethnicity, gender, and religion/spirituality as doorways to understanding how culture and values may intersect with systems of care

Film: *What Matters to Families: Speaking the Same Language, Initiative for Pediatric Palliative Care*

Readings on class:

Kirchhoff, L. S. (2003). Case study of Milton, "the cowboy." *Smith College Studies in Social Work, 73,* 463–478.

Williams, B. R. (2004). Dying young, dying poor: A sociological examination of existential suffering among low-socioeconomic status patients. *Journal of Palliative Care, 7,* 27–37.

Readings on ethnicity:

Blackhall, L. J., Frank, G., Murphy, S. T., Michel, V., Palmer, J. M., & Azen, S. P. (1999). Ethnicity and attitudes towards life sustaining technology. *Social Science and Medicine, 48*(12), 1779–1789.

Kagaway-Singer, M., & Blackhall, L. J. (2001). Negotiating cross-cultural issues at the end of life: "You got to go where he lives." *Journal of the American Medical Association, 286*(23), 2993–3001.

Readings on gender:

McGoldrick, M. (2004). Gender and mourning. In F. Walsh & M. McGoldrick (Eds.), *Living beyond loss: Death in the family* (pp. 99–118). New York: W. W. Norton.

Noppe, I. C. (2004). Gender and death: Parallel and intersecting pathways. In Berzoff & Silverman, pp. 206–225.

Readings on religion and spirituality:

Clarfield, A. M., Gordon, M., Markwell, H., & Alibhai, S. M. H. (2003). Ethical issues in end-of-life geriatric care: The approach of three monotheistic religions—Judaism, Catholicism, and Islam. *Journal of the American Geriatrics Society, 51,* 1149–1154.

Jacobs, C. (2004). Spirituality and end-of-life care practice for social workers. In Berzoff & Silverman, pp. 188–205.

Session 3 Assessment from a family perspective

Objective: To identify basic components of assessing family dynamics in situations of critical illness

Film: *What Matters to Families: Big Choices, Little Choices, Initiative for Pediatric Palliative Care*

Reading:

Farber, S., Egnew, T., & Farber, A. (2004). What is respectful death? In Berzoff & Silverman, pp. 102–127.

Kissane & Bloch, chapters 1–5, 7

Klass, D. (1999). Developing a cross-cultural model of grief: The state of the field. *Omega: Journal of Death and Dying, 39*(3), 153–178.

Clinical Assessment across the Life Span: Understanding the Developmental Needs of Children, Adults, and Elders

Session 4 Families caring for a critically ill child

Objective: To identify developmental concerns for families caring for critically ill children, and strategies for effective social work practice

Film: *What Matters to Families: Knowing Who We Are, Initiative for Pediatric Palliative Care*

Reading:

Institute of Medicine. (2003). Pathways to a child's death. In *When children die: Improving palliative and end-of-life care for children and their families* (pp. 72–103). Washington, DC: National Academy Press.

Jones, B., & Weisenfluh, S. (2003). Pediatric palliative care and end-of-life care: Developmental and spiritual issues of dying children. *Smith College Studies in Social Work, 73*(3), 423–443.

Session 5 Families caring for a critically ill adult
Objective: To identify midlife developmental concerns using two case studies: a gay couple facing critical illness, and a physician with end-stage heart failure

Film: *Silverlake Life: The View from Here*

Reading:
His, S. D. (2004). *Closing the chart: A dying physician examines family, faith and medicine.* Albuquerque: University of New Mexico Press.
Thompson, B., & Colon, Y. (2004). Lesbians and gay men at the end of their lives: Psychosocial concerns. In Berzoff & Silverman, pp. 482–498.
Werner-Lin, A., & Moro, T. (2004). Unacknowledged and stigmatized losses. In F. Walsh & M. McGoldrick (Eds.), *Living beyond loss: Death in the family* (pp. 245–271). New York: W. W. Norton.

Session 6 Families caring for a critically ill elder
Objective: To explore dynamics related to ageism and how this affects end-of-life decision making

Film: *Dying at Grace*

Reading:
Kutzen, H., & Lindhorst, T. (1996). What to expect as the end of life approaches. In *End of life: Information for caregivers* [Brochure]. New Orleans, LA: Delta Region AIDS Education and Training Center.
Moss, M. S., & Moss, S. Z. (1989). Death of the very old. In K. J. Doka (Ed.), *Disenfranchised grief: Recognizing hidden sorrow* (pp. 213–227). Lexington, MA: Lexington Books.
Quill, chapters 6, 7, 8

Social Work Practice Skills: Effective Work within Fragmented Systems of Care

Session 7 Decision-making conferences
Objective: To identify dynamics in interprofessional team meetings and to understand social work roles and skills in these meetings

Film: *Survival Run* (deep relationship building)

Reading:

Ambuel, B. (2000). Conducting a family conference. *Principles and Practice of Supportive Oncology, 3*(3), 1–12.

Rabow, M. W., Hauser, J. M., & Adams, J. (2004). Supporting family caregivers at the end of life: "They don't know what they don't know." *Journal of the American Medical Association, 291,* 483–491.

Zilberfein, F., & Hurwitz, E. (2003). Clinical social work practice at the end of life. *Smith College Studies in Social Work, 73*(3), 299–324.

Session 8 Palliative care in prisions

Objective: To understand how work in prison settings with the terminally ill informs our understanding of social work advocacy in complex systems

Film: *Angola Prison Hospice*

Reading:

Enders, S. R. (2004). End-of-life care in the prison system: Implications for social work. In Berzoff & Silverman, pp. 609–627.

Granse, B. L. (2003). Why should we even care? Hospice social work practice in a prison setting. *Smith College Studies in Social Work, 7*(3), 359–376.

Session 9 Relentless self-care

Objective: Exploring our own understanding of suffering and service by reflecting on how we care for ourselves while giving care to others

Reading:

Browning, D. (2004). Fragments of love: Explorations in the ethnography of suffering and professional caregiving. In Berzoff & Silverman, pp. 21–42.

Ostaseski, F. (1996). Exploring our intention in service. *Alternative Therapies in Health and Medicine, 2*(3).

Session 10 Making meaning of endings

Objective: To reflect on endings and meaning making in the context of end-of-life care

Film: *A Family Undertaking: Home Funerals in America*

Reading:

Breitbart, W., Gibson, C., Poppito, S. R., & Berg, A. (2004). Psychotherapeutic interventions at the end of life: A focus on meaning and spirituality. *Canadian Journal of Psychiatry, 49*(6), 366–372.

Puchalski, C. M. (2002). Spirituality. In A. M. Berger, R. K. Portenoy, & D. E. Weissman (Eds.), *Principles and practice of palliative care and supportive oncology* (2nd ed., pp. 799–812). Philadelphia: Lippincott Williams & Wilkins.

21

Death and Dying
Issues across the Life Span

Sara Sanders

COURSE DESCRIPTION

Students enrolled in this course will be examining issues of death, dying, grief, and loss in an experiential fashion. The course is specifically designed to introduce students to the field of end-of-life care by assisting them in confronting many of their own concerns about the death, dying, and grieving process. It examines the historical, cultural, societal, and personal perspectives on death and dying in modern society. The course will introduce students to the following topics: (1) cultural and historical perspectives on death and dying, as well as grief and loss; (2) reactions to death and dying among children, adolescents, adults, and older adults; (3) theoretical premises related to death and dying; (4) issues related to personal death anxiety and death phobia and strategies to address these issues; (5) coping mechanisms and self-care strategies of professionals who work in the field; (6) the roles of different professionals who work in the death-and-dying field; and (7) issues related to grief, loss, and bereavement.

OBJECTIVES

The goal of this course is:

- To provide an overview of the theoretical premises associated with death, dying, and grief in modern society, specifically the work of Alan Wolfelt, Pauline Boss, and Elisabeth Kübler-Ross
- To present a historical analysis for current views and beliefs about death and dying
- To examine issues related to death and dying based on age, specifically focusing on children, adolescents, middle-aged adults, and older adults
- To identify cultural differences in reactions to death and dying

- To provide students with a hands-on experience in confronting their own fears about death and dying by examining personal issues associated with death and dying, including death phobia and death anxiety, and identifying strategies that can be used to address personal death anxiety
- To introduce students to service providers who work within the field of death and dying, including social workers, nurses, funeral directors, coroners, and pathologists
- To identify resources that are needed by families who are dealing with death-and-dying issues, including funeral planning, advance directive, autopsies, organ donation, hospice care, and therapy
- To introduce students to basic intervention strategies to use with dying patients and their families, such as play therapy, grief therapy, reminiscence, and support groups

By the end of the course, students will be able to:

- Identify the major theoretical premises driving the field of death and dying
- Provide information on the historical issues that have influenced current perspectives on death and dying
- Contrast the various ways different cultural and racial groups address death and dying
- Apply strategies to assess and intervene with children, adolescents, middle-aged adults, and older adults facing death and dying
- Identify personal areas of death anxiety and death phobia and strategies to address these issues
- Recognize the roles of different service providers who work within the death-and-dying field
- Identify the types of decisions that families must make when confronted with death and dying and the types of services that are available to assist them with these decisions
- Recognize the different types of options that may be considered by dying individuals with their family members, including hospice/palliative care, advance directives, and assisted suicide

INSTRUCTIONAL METHODS

This course will be taught using lectures, discussion, audio-visuals, guest speakers, projects, readings, papers, exams, class presentations, and role-playing.

REQUIRED TEXTS

Callanan, M., & Kelley, P. (1992). *Final gifts: Understanding the special awareness, needs and communications of the dying*. New York: Bantam Books.

DeSpelder, L. A., & Strickland, A. L. (2002). *The last dance: Encountering death and dying* (6th ed.). Boston: McGraw-Hill.

COURSE REQUIREMENTS

Death-and-dying interviews: Students will be conducting a series of interviews in order to obtain a deeper understanding of the diverse views of the death-and-dying process. The interviews need to be conducted with four individuals: one who is eighteen or younger, one who is between nineteen and forty, one who is between forty-one and sixty-four, and one who is sixty-five or older. It is best if these individuals are not immediate family members. The interviews need to cover the following topics:

The interviewees' views of the dying process

Where they learned about death and dying

What their culture/religion states about the dying process

What they believe happens after one dies

What they would do if they learned they had one month to live

If they could, they how they would plan their funeral

How they want to be remembered

Additionally, students should give an assessment of the strengths that the person could draw on when faced with a death-and-dying situation, as well as potential problems that could develop when he or she is faced with a death-and-dying experience. In this paper, students should consider how development stage may be affecting each individual's view of death. This paper should be ten to twelve pages long. For MSW/MA and PhD students, this paper needs to be fifteen pages and should include an analysis of the interviews integrating theory and culture. Students are also encouraged to consider areas in the interview that may require future intervention or could be used as strengths that could be drawn on by a health-care professional if a death in the family system occurred.

Personal statement paper: For this paper, students are asked to examine their own views of the dying process by utilizing the questions above (from the interview paper). Additionally, students should include an analysis of their first experience with the death-and-dying process, specifically examining how the experience affected them and their family, and what services they wish they could have had provided to assist with the grieving process. This paper should be eight pages in length.

Analysis of Five Wishes exercise: For this assignment, students should discuss their Five Wishes assignment with at least two family members. Students should specifically define the assignment and their wishes and should then discuss with these two family members their wishes at the end of life and any types of plans that they have made for an unexpected illness or death. For this paper, students should write a reflection of this conversation and its impact not only on themselves but on the family members they discussed it with. This paper should be five pages long.

Examinations: There will be two take-home examinations in this course. The examinations will be based on case studies and other global questions discussed in lecture and by guest speakers.

COURSE OUTLINE

Session 1
Introduction
DeSpelder & Strickland, chapter 1
Attitudes toward death
The meaning of death
Defining death in our modern world
Film: *Living with Dying*

Session 2
DeSpelder & Strickland, chapter 2
Historical and cultural analysis of death and dying
Examination of African American, Latino, and Asian death customs
Film: *A Different Kind of Care* (Moyers)

Session 3
DeSpelder & Strickland, chapter 3
Sociocultural influences of our attitudes on death
Exercise: Examination of children's movies for hidden messages about death (*The Lion King, Snow White,* and *Finding Nemo*)

Session 4
DeSpelder & Strickland, chapter 4
End-of-life issues in health-care settings
Issues of ethics, dying in an institutional setting, pain control, and pharmacology
Speaker: Hospice provider

Session 5
DeSpelder & Strickland, chapter 5
Callanan & Kelley, pp. 1–63
Living as a dying individual
Self-reflections on living each day facing death
Film: *Tuesdays with Morrie*

Session 6
DeSpelder & Strickland, chapter 6
Callanan & Kelley, pp. 69–134

Ethical decisions as we face the end of our lives
Examination of the dying process (biological, social, spiritual, and psychological changes that occur as a person begins the active dying process)

Session 7 DeSpelder & Strickland, chapter 8
Callanan & Kelley, pp. 141–237
Planning for our deaths (dealing with funerals, obituaries, and cremation)
Exercise: Students are asked to plan their own funerals and write their own obituaries. These will be shared in class.
Field trip: Funeral home

Session 8 DeSpelder & Strickland, chapter 9
Laws and death
Powers of attorney, advance directives
State laws about death status
Organ donation
Exercise: Pass out Five Wishes booklet in class for students to discuss in groups and then individually complete. Have students share how they completed the booklet and the motivation for their end-of-life decisions.

Session 9 DeSpelder & Strickland, chapters 7 and 10
Understanding grief and loss
Working with dying children and children who are grieving
Film: *Talking with Children about Death* (Mr. Rogers)

Session 10 DeSpelder & Strickland, chapter 11
Adults and death
Issues facing widows and widowers
Issues facing parents who have lost a child

Session 11 DeSpelder & Strickland, chapter 12
Sudden death
Issues following suicide and murder
Euthanasia and Oregon's law on physician-assisted suicide
Film: *A Death of One's Own* (Moyers)

Session 12 DeSpelder & Strickland, chapter 13
Mass fatalities: Natural and human-made disasters
Communicable diseases
Speaker: Medical examiner's office and forensic pathologist

Session 13 DeSpelder & Strickland, chapter 14
Spirituality and the end of life

Near-death experiences
Use of spirituality in counseling dying individuals and their families
Speaker: Panel of individuals from different faith backgrounds

Session 14 DeSpelder & Strickland, chapter 15
End-of-life issues in the future
Death education
Film: *A Time to Change* (Moyers)

22

Death and Dying
Implications and Challenges for Practice

Tracy Schroepfer

COURSE DESCRIPTION

Death and Dying: Implications and Challenges for Practice is an elective course that focuses on social work practice with children, adolescents, adults, and elders who have a terminal illness, as well as their families.

COURSE OVERVIEW

This three-part course is designed to provide the knowledge base and practice skills necessary for working effectively with terminally ill individuals of all ages and their families. In part 1, background information is provided on the shifting patterns of death and dying throughout American history, the theories constructed to assist professionals caring for terminally ill individuals, the various end-of-life models of care, and the many cultural approaches to dying and death. In part 2, students are provided with opportunities via readings, discussions, and exercises to develop self-awareness of the values and beliefs they hold toward dying and death. This self-awareness will allow them to work more effectively with terminally ill individuals and their families. Part 3 covers knowledge and practice skills regarding the assessment and fulfillment of the psychosocial needs of children, adolescents, adults, and elders who have a terminal illness, as well as their families. Issues specific to each age population are discussed, as well as those of special-needs populations such as terminally ill individuals who have a developmental disability, a mental illness, or AIDS. Information is also provided regarding final planning for dying and death, practice skills for mediating and facilitating such planning with terminally ill individuals and their families, and overarching ethical and moral dilemmas that may arise.

OBJECTIVES

This course will provide students with the knowledge and skills necessary for their professional development in providing terminally ill individuals and their families with quality end-of-life care. More specifically, students will:

- Acquire knowledge of the legal and financial issues related to death and dying
- Acquire knowledge of the history of death and dying in the United States and an understanding of the implications for practice and policy
- Acquire knowledge of different models of end-of-life care and relevant theories
- Acquire knowledge of other cultures' beliefs and rituals surrounding dying and death
- Develop an awareness of their own assumptions, beliefs, values, and behaviors with regard to the dying process, death, grief, and their own mortality
- Develop a deeper awareness of how these beliefs and values may influence their assessment of others' behavior and situations, and ethical dilemmas that may result
- Develop an understanding and awareness regarding the role discrimination, economic deprivation, oppression, power differentials, and social inequalities can play in the dying process
- Develop an awareness of ethical issues and dilemmas related to death and dying
- Develop the appropriate communication skills necessary for discussing end-of-life issues with terminally ill children, adolescents, adults, elders, and their families, as well as special populations such as terminally ill individuals who are developmentally disabled, have a chronic mental illness, or have AIDS
- Develop skills for effectively assessing the psychosocial and spiritual needs of terminally ill individuals and their families
- Acquire the knowledge and skills necessary to assist and empower terminally ill individuals and their families throughout the dying process
- Develop skills for identifying and locating resources for terminally ill individuals
- Develop decision-making and mediation skills necessary to assist terminally ill individuals and their families
- Develop the interpersonal and group skills necessary for working on interdisciplinary teams

COURSE OUTLINE

Part 1

Session 1 Introductions
Overview of course, syllabus, and grading
Goals of dying-and-death education

Session 2 History of dying and death in the United States
Dying trajectories
Location of death
Legal issues and self-determination
Social work's growing role

Reading:

Bern-Klug, M., Gessert, C., & Forbes, S. (2001). The need to revise assumptions about the end of life: Implications for social work practice. *Health and Social Work, 26*(1), 38–48.

Callanan, M., & Kelley, P. (1992). We must go to the park. In *Final Gifts* (pp. 141–149). New York: Simon and Schuster.

Gostin, L. O. (1997). Deciding life and death in the courtroom: From Quinlan to Cruzan, Glucksberg, and Vacco—a brief history and analysis of constitutional protection of the "right to die." *Journal of the American Medical Association, 78*(18), 1523–1528.

Luptak, M. (2004). Social work and end-of-life care for older people: A historical perspective. *Health and Social Work, 29*(1), 7–15.

Walter, T. (1996). Facing death without tradition. In G. Howarth & P. Jupp (Eds.), *Contemporary issues in the sociology of death, dying, and disposal* (pp. 193–204). New York: St. Martin's Press.

Session 3 Coping with dying and death: Theoretical approaches
End-of-life theories
Integrating theory into clinical practice

Reading:

Bern-Klug, M. (2004). The ambiguous dying syndrome. *Health and Social Work, 29*(1), 55–65.

Corr, C. A. (1991–1992). A task-based approach to coping with dying. *Omega: Journal of Death and Dying, 24*(2), 81–94.

Glaser, B. G., & Strauss, A. L. (1964). Awareness contexts and social interaction. *American Sociological Review, 29*(5), 669–679.

Kübler-Ross, E. (1970). The care of the dying: Whose job is it? *Psychiatry in Medicine, 1*(2), 103–107.

Session 4 End-of-life models of care
Definitions
Goals
Strengths and limitations
Role of health-care professionals

Reading:

Finke, B., Bowannie, T., & Kitzes, J. (2004). Palliative care in the pueblo of Zuni. *Journal of Palliative Medicine, 7*(1), 135–143.

National Hospice Workgroup. (2003, March–April). Access to hospice care: Expanding boundaries, overcoming barriers. *Hastings Center Report,* pp. S6–S12.

Stein, G. (2004). Improving our care at life's end: Making a difference. *Health and Social Work, 29*(1), 77–79.

Von Guten, C. F. (2002). Secondary and tertiary palliative care in US hospitals. *Journal of the American Medical Association, 287*(7), 875–881.

Zerzan, J., Stearns, S., & Hanson, L. (2000). Access to palliative care and hospice in nursing homes. *Journal of the American Medical Association, 284*(19), 2489–2494.

Session 5 Term paper topics must be approved by this date.
Cultural beliefs and rituals surrounding dying and death
Awareness and acknowledgement and respect
Attitudes toward death
Death-related practices
Ethical dilemmas

Reading:

Barham, D. (2003). The last 48 hours of life: A case study of symptom control for a patient taking a Buddhist approach to dying. *International Journal of Palliative Nursing, 9*(6), 245–251.

Born, W., Greiner, K. A., Greiner, M. D., Sylvia, E., Butler, J., & Ahluwalia, J. S. (2004). Knowledge, attitudes, and beliefs about end-of-life care among inner-city African Americans and Latinos. *Journal of Palliative Medicine, 7*(2), 247–256.

Cort, M. A. (2004). Cultural mistrust and use of hospice care: Challenges and remedies. *Journal of Palliative Medicine, 7*(1), 63–71.

Kagawa-Singer, M., & Blackhall, L. J. (2001). Negotiating cross-cultural issues at the end of life: "You got to go where he lives." *Journal of the American Medical Association, 286*(23), 2993–3001.

Part 2

Session 6 Journal entries for weeks 2–5 due
Coping with dying and death: The professional (part 1)
Beliefs, values, and behaviors
Self-awareness
Ethical dilemmas and implications
Boundary setting

Reading:

Abramson, M. (1996). Reflections on knowing oneself ethically: Toward a working framework for social work practice. *Families in Society, 77*(4), 195–201.

Mattison, M. (2000). Ethical decision-making: The person in the process. *Social Work, 45*(3), 201–212.

Reamer, F. G. (2003). Boundary issues in social work: Managing dual relationships. *Social Work, 48*(1), 121–133.

Ross, E. K. (2000). What is it like to be dying? *American Journal of Nursing, 100*(10), 96AA, 96CC, 96EE, 96GG–96II.

Session 7 Obituary due
Coping with dying and death: The professional (part 2)
Professional power differentials
Caring for oneself
Professionals caring for professionals

Reading:

Itzhaky, H., & Lipschitz-Elhawi, R. (2004). Hope as a strategy in supervising social workers of terminally ill patients. *Health and Social Work, 29*(1), 46–54.

Poulin, J. E., & Walter, C. A. (1993). Burnout in gerontological social work. *Social Work, 38*(3), 305–310.

Reese, D. J., & Sontag, M. (2001). Successful interpersonal collaboration on the hospice team. *Health and Social Work, 26*(3), 167–175.

Roy, D. J. (2003). The wounded bird . . . a meditation on fragility. *Journal of Palliative Care, 19*(2), 75–76.

Strug, D., & Podell, C. (2002). A bereavement support group for pediatric HIV/AIDS case managers and social workers: Helping members cope with dying children. *Social Work with Groups, 25*(3), 61–75.

Thiedke, C. C. (2000). Grieving the death of a patient. *Family Practice Management, 7*(5), 78.

Part 3

Session 8 Thesis statements due
The dying experience
Physical symptoms
Psychosocial symptoms
Pain management
Signs and symptoms of active dying

Reading:

Chochinov, H. M. (2002). Dignity-conserving care—a new model for palliative care: Helping the patient feel valued. *Journal of the American Medical Association, 87*(17), 2253–2260.

Furman, J. (2004). Healing the mind and spirit as the body fails. *Nursing, 34*(4), 50–51.

Mendenhall, M. (2003). Psychosocial aspects of pain management: A conceptual framework for social workers on pain management teams. *Social Work in Health Care, 36*(4), 35–51.

Rumbold, B. D. (2003). Caring for the spirit: Lessons from working with the dying. *Medical Journal of Australia, 179*(6), S11–S13.

Staton, J., Shuy, R., & Byock, I. (2001). The final days of life. In *A few months to live: Different paths to life's end* (pp. 271–288). Washington, DC: Georgetown University Press.

Session 9 Psychosocial assessment
Person-in-environment approach
Identifying psychological stressors and mental health issues
Identifying therapeutic goals and steps for preparing for death
Identifying spiritual needs
Resource acquisition
Empowering terminally ill individuals and family members
Advocacy

Reading:

Armes, P. J., & Addington-Hall, J. M. (2003). Perspectives on symptom control in patients receiving community palliative care. *Palliative Medicine, 17,* 608–615.

Block, S. (2000). Assessing and managing depression in the terminally ill patient. *Annals of Internal Medicine, 132,* 209–218.

Block, S. D. (2001). Psychological considerations, growth, and transcendence at the end of life: The art of the possible. *Journal of the American Medical Association, 285*(22), 2898–2904.

Pessin, H., Rosenfeld, B., & Breitbart, W. (2002). Assessing psychological distress near the end of life. *American Behavioral Scientist, 46*(3), 357–372.

Werth, J. L., Gordon, J. R., & Johnson, R. R. (2002). Psychosocial issues near the end of life. *Aging and Mental Health, 6*(4), 402–412.

Session 10 Children, adolescents, and family
Death-related concepts and attitudes
Coping with terminal illness
Communicating and assisting

Reading:

Browning, D. (2004). To show our humanness: Relational and communicative competence in pediatric palliative care. *Bioethics Forum, 18*(3/4), 23–28.

Davies, B., Brenner, P., Orloff, S., Sumner, L., & Worden, W. (2002). Addressing spirituality in pediatric hospice and palliative care. *Journal of Palliative Care, 18*(1), 59–67.

Freyer, D. R. (2004). Care of the dying adolescent: Special considerations. *Pediatrics, 113*(2), 381–388.

Himelstein, B. P., Hilden, J. M., Boldt, A. M., & Weissman, D. (2004). Pediatric palliative care. *New England of Journal Medicine, 350*(17), 1752–1762.

Stillion, J. M., & Papadatou, D. (2002). Suffer the children. *American Behavioral Scientist, 46*(2), 299–315.

Session 11 Journal entries for weeks 6–10 due
Adults and elders and family
Death-related concepts and attitudes
Coping with terminal illness
Communicating and assisting

Reading:

Ajaj, A., Singh, M. P., & Abdulla, A. J. J. (2001). Should elder patients be told they have cancer? Questionnaire survey of older people. *British Medical Journal, 323,* 1160.

Hudson, P. L., Aranda, S., & Kristjanson, L. J. (2004). Meeting the supportive needs of family caregivers in palliative care: Challenges for health professionals. *Journal of Palliative Medicine, 7*(1), 19–25.

Hui-Mei, A., & Lin, H. (2003). Factors related to attitudes toward death among American and Chinese older adults. *Omega: Journal of Death and Dying, 47*(1), 3–23.

Sheehan, D., & Schirm, V. (2003). End-of-life care of older adults. *American Journal of Nursing, 103*(11), 48–58.

Vig, E. K., & Pearlman, R. A. (2004). Good and bad dying from the perspective of terminally ill men. *Archives of Internal Medicine, 164*(9), 977–981.

Weinrich, M. D., Curtis, J. R., Shannon, S. E., Carline, J. D., Ambrozy, D. M., & Ramsey, P. G. (2001). Communicating with dying patients within the spectrum of medical care from terminal diagnosis to death. *Archives of Internal Medicine, 161*(6), 868–874.

Session 12 Terminally ill individuals with special needs and their families
Developmental disability
Mental illness
HIV/AIDS
Dementia

Reading:

Foti, M. E., Okun, S. N., Wogrin, C., & Corbeil, Y. J. (2003). *End-of-life care for persons with serious mental illness: The curriculum for mental health providers.* Massachusetts Department of Mental Health, Metro Suburban Area.

Freidman, R. I. (1998). Use of advance directives: Facilitating health care decisions by adults with mental retardation and their families. *Mental Retardation, 36*(6), 444–456.

Gessert, C. E., Forbes, S., & Bern-Klug, M. (2000–2001). Planning end-of-life care for patients with dementia: Roles of families and health professionals. *Omega: Journal of Death and Dying, 42*(4), 273–291.

Ruiz, P. (2000). Living and dying with HIV: A psychosocial perspective. *American Journal of Psychiatry, 157*(1), 110–113.

Todd, S. (2002). Death does not become us: The absence of death and dying in intellectual disability research. *Journal of Gerontological Social Work, 38*(1/2), 225–238.

Wenger, N. S., Kanouse, D. E., Collins, R. L., Liu, H., Schuster, M. A., Gifford, A. L., et al. (2001). End-of-life discussions and preferences among persons with HIV. *Journal of the American Medical Association, 285*(22), 2880–2887.

Session 13 Helping patients and family through the grieving process
Grieving in the dying process
Survivors' grief

Reading:

Hurley, A. C., & Volicer, L. (2002). Alzheimer disease: "It's okay, Mama, if you want to go, it's okay." *Journal of the American Medical Association, 288*(18), 2324–2332.

Luchterhand, C. (1998). What is unique for adults with mental retardation? In *Helping adults with mental retardation grieve a death loss* (pp. 15–40). Philadelphia: Accelerated Development.

Nenner, F. (2002). The knapsack. *Journal of the American Medical Association, 287*(4), 417–418.

Saldinger, A., Cain, A., & Porterfield, K. (2003). Managing traumatic stress in children anticipating parental death. *Psychiatry, 66*(2), 168–179.

Session 14 Term paper due
Ethical issues
Confidentiality, autonomy, and self-determination
Withdrawing or withholding treatment
Terminal sedation
Physician-assisted suicide and physician-assisted euthanasia
Moral dilemmas

Reading:

Anonymous. (2002). Client self-determination in end-of-life decisions. *American Behavioral Scientist, 46*(3), 434–438.

Cohen, L. M., Germain, M. J., & Poppel, D. M. (2003). Practical considerations in dialysis withdrawal: "To have that option is a blessing." *Journal of the American Medical Association, 289*(16), 2113–2119.

Lavery, J. V., Boyle, J., Dickens, B. M., Maclean, H., & Singer, P. A. (2001). Origins of the desire for euthanasia and assisted suicide in people with HIV-1 or AIDS: A qualitative study. *The Lancet, 358*(9279), 362–367.

Manetta, A. A., & Wells, J. G. (2001). Ethical issues in the social worker's role in physician-assisted suicide. *Health and Social Work, 26*(3), 160–166.

Quill, T. E., & Byock, I. R. (2000). Responding to intractable terminal suffering: The role of terminal sedation and voluntary refusal of food and fluids. *Annals of Internal Medicine, 132*(5), 408–414.

Werner, P., Carmel, S., & Ziedenberg, H. (2004). Nurses' and social workers' attitudes and beliefs about and involvement in life-sustaining treatment decisions. *Health and Social Work, 29*(1), 27–35.

Session 15 Advance directive due
Journal entries for weeks 11–14 and final entry due
Final plans
Advance directives
Organ donation
Inheritance
Memorials and funerals

Reading:

Briggs, L. (2003). Shifting the focus of advance care planning: Using an in-depth interview to build and strengthen relationships. *Innovations in End-of-Life Care, 5*(2), 1–16. Available at www.edc.org/lastacts

Carson, N. (2003). *Conversations before the crisis.* Washington, DC: Last Acts National Program Office.

Hobart, K. R. (2001). Death and dying and the social work role. *Journal of Gerontological Social Work, 36*(3/4), 181–192.

Stum, M. S. (2003). *Tips for planning ahead.* St. Paul: University of Minnesota Extension Service.

METHODS OF EVALUATION

Weekly journal: A key goal of this course is to provide you with a deeper awareness and understanding of your own values and beliefs regarding dying and death. In addition to increasing your awareness and understanding, it is also important that you recognize how these values and beliefs may influence your assessment of and relations with terminally ill clients and their families.

To assist you in gaining this awareness and understanding, each week you will be expected to reflect on and respond to the weekly readings and class discussions by journaling your thoughts, reactions, and concerns. Please type your journal using the written assignment policy below. You must generate at least a full page and a half per week. Your final entry should include your thoughts on the following: (1) how this class has increased your awareness of the values and beliefs you hold toward the process of dying and death; (2) how you feel these values and beliefs might affect your assessment of, and relation with, clients, families, and fellow staff members; and (3) the ethical dilemmas you might face as a result of value and belief differences.

You may earn up to five points each time you turn in your journal. You will not be graded on the content of the journal since the purpose of a journal is to express your thoughts freely. Your grade will be based on whether your journal is turned in on time and whether you have followed the instructions above.

Reaction papers: Undergraduate students are required to write four reaction papers, each based on one reading chosen from weeks 3 through 15; each reading must be from a different week. In these papers you should critically evaluate what you have read and respond by discussing the following: (1) your overall reaction to the reading, including new questions the reading raised for you, and how it did or did not expand your knowledge and understanding of the overall topic; (2) your feelings regarding the reading's strengths and weaknesses; and (3) how the reading serves to inform social work practice or policy. These reaction papers are to be two to three pages long.

Graduate students are required to write four reaction papers based on four different sets of readings chosen from weeks 3 through 15. Each paper should synthesize and critically evaluate the chosen readings by addressing the following: (1) your overall reaction to the week's readings, including new questions the readings raised for you, and how they did or did not expand your knowledge and understanding of the overall topic; (2) your feelings regarding the readings' strengths and weaknesses; and (3) how the readings serve to inform social work practice or policy. These reaction papers are to be three to four pages long.

Obituary: For this assignment, you will be given an instructional sheet with the general areas you are to cover.

Advance directive: You will be required to complete an advance directive document.

Term paper: Undergraduate students will be required to write a paper on an issue pertinent to the practice of social work in end-of-life care. In your paper, you should discuss (1) background information on the issue and how it evolved; (2) relevance of the issue to social work practice; (3) the role oppression, economic deprivation, or discrimination plays; (4) relevant social work practices or policies; (5) potential ethical dilemmas; and (6) recommendations for addressing this issue within the realm of social work practice. You may not use articles or book chapters assigned to you for this course as reference materials for your paper, nor any newspaper or magazine articles. Your sources should come from journals and books (social work and non–social work), and you should use APA style to cite the author, title, and source. Undergraduate term papers should be between six and twelve pages long, and graduate term papers between twelve and fifteen pages long.

Part Seven

MSW Syllabi: Loss, Grief, and Bereavement

23

Therapeutic Approaches to Loss and Change

Dorothy S. Becvar

COURSE DESCRIPTION

In this course, therapeutic approaches to various kinds of loss and change are examined. Emphasis is placed on understanding the grief responses to such events in the personal lives, families, and workplaces of social workers and those they serve. Current literature, research, media, and other resources will be used to investigate the impact and ramifications of loss-and-change experiences, as well as ways to help both social workers and their clients deal with these experiences. These experiences may be associated with individual and family developmental processes as well as major life events in the realms of relationships, jobs, homes, physical capacity, group memberships, respect, trust, self-esteem, dying, and death.

OBJECTIVES

At the conclusion of this course, each student will be able to:

- Demonstrate understanding of the range of experiences of change that may elicit a grief response in oneself as well as others
- Demonstrate understanding of age-related changes and losses throughout the life cycle, including the various factors that may influence individual responses to them
- Demonstrate knowledge of the patterns and characteristics of grieving in children and adults relative to the various kinds of loss and change they may experience
- Demonstrate knowledge of the complex ethical and legal questions and choices that have arisen in conjunction with technological advances in the medical realm
- Demonstrate comprehension of ways to support the dying process and to facilitate a good death

- Demonstrate comprehension of appropriate ways to work with and support those living in the presence of grief related to the experience of the full range of loss-and-change experiences

TEACHING AND LEARNING METHODS

This course uses didactic instruction, large and small group discussions, film presentations, role plays, and simulations as appropriate. Students are expected to be active participants in the teaching/learning process and to recognize and share responsibility both for their own learning and for that of their classmates.

REQUIRED TEXT

Becvar, D. S. (2001). *In the presence of grief: Helping family members successfully resolve death, dying and bereavement issues.* New York: Guilford Press.

METHODS OF EVALUATION

1. Students will complete all assignments on schedule and come to class on time and prepared to participate fully in discussions of the readings and in all other class activities.
2. Students will keep a journal of reactions, reflections, and questions related to activities and experiences both in and outside the classroom. Journals will be due on a biweekly basis.
3. Students will complete several short essays:

   Assignment #1—Personal Reflections: Students will complete four instruments (Perspectives on Dying Personal Questionnaire, Personal Timeline; Thinking about Your Life, Your Dying, and Your Death; Life Events Inventory) aimed at assessing the losses and changes they have experienced in their own lives, their coping strategies and abilities, their perspectives on death and dying in general, and their beliefs about their own living and dying in particular.

   Assignment #2—Interviews and Experiences: Students will participate in six activities chosen from the following list—three interviews and three experiences—and write brief summaries for each activity chosen.

   - Visit a hospice
   - Visit a cemetery
   - Visit a funeral home
   - Visit the coroner's office
   - Volunteer on a suicide hotline

- Volunteer in a homeless shelter
- Interview someone who has experienced a divorce
- Interview someone who has experienced job loss or homelessness
- Interview someone who has had a close brush with death
- Interview someone who has lost a loved one through death
- Interview an elderly person about aging and dying
- Interview someone from a different culture on his or her perspectives on death

Assignment #3—Analysis of a Major Loss: Students will briefly describe the events surrounding a major loss in their own lives. In part 1 of the paper, this is to be done in the form of a narrative or story of the loss. Students should describe the feelings experienced, what people did to try to help, and what people said or did that made things worse, as well as how long ago the events occurred, the student's age at the time and his or her feelings then about the loss as well as subsequent experiences related to it. In part 2, this same loss is to be analyzed as if it happened to someone else, using the third person and thinking as a social worker working with someone who has experienced this loss, and making reference to either or both of the texts as well as related information as appropriate.

4. Working in small groups, students will pick a topic related to an experience of loss and/or change to explore in depth. All topics must be approved by the instructor. Students will then prepare both a paper and a class presentation on their topic. In both the paper and the presentation they will be expected to go beyond the level and scope of class readings, discussions, and texts and provide information about therapeutic approaches and appropriate resources for dealing with the issue. The paper is to be typed and double spaced and must use APA format. As part of their presentation, students should examine concepts, issues, and dilemmas related to the topic through the use of films.
5. Students will evaluate their own work as well as that of the other members of their group based on the following criteria:

   - Attendence: How often did the student attend classes and other small group meetings?
   - Participation: To what degree did the student involve him- or herself in group discussions and decision making?
   - Contribution: How well did the student fulfill his or her commitment to the group's goals and requirements?

COURSE OUTLINE

Session 1 Introductions
The nature of loss and change

Session 2 Psychological losses from youth to old age
Assignment #1 due

Reading:

Scott-Maxwell, F. (1968). *The measure of my days.* New York: Penguin (pp. 5–57).

Viorst, J. (1986). *Necessary losses: The loves, illusions, dependencies, and impossible expectations that all of us have to give up in order to grow.* New York: Simon and Schuster (pp. 21–80).

Session 3 Journal #1 due

Session 4 Understanding death, dying, and bereavement

Reading:

Becvar, chapters 1 and 2

Becvar, D. S. (2003). The impact on the family therapist of a focus on death, dying and bereavement. *Journal of Marital and Family Therapy, 29*(4), 469–477.

Session 5 When death comes unannounced
Journal #2 due

Reading:

Becvar, chapter 3

Dunne, E. J., & Dunne-Maxim, K. (2004). Working with families in the aftermath of suicide. In F. Walsh & M. McGoldrick (Eds.), *Living beyond loss: Death in the family* (2nd ed., pp. 272–284). New York: Guilford Press.

Session 6 When death is anticipated
Assignment #2 due

Reading:

Becvar, chapter 4

Wright, K. (2003). Relationships with death: The terminally ill talk about dying. *Journal of Marital and Family Therapy, 29*(4), 439–453.

Session 7 When the question of euthanasia emerges
Journal #3 due

Reading:

Becvar, chapter 5

Rolland, J. S. (2004). Helping families with anticipatory loss and terminal illness. In F. Walsh & M. McGoldrick (Eds.), *Living beyond loss: Death in the family* (2nd ed., pp. 213–236). New York: Guilford Press.

Session 8 When a child dies

Reading:

Becvar, chapter 6

Nader, K. O. (1997). Treating traumatic grief in systems. In C. R. Figley, B. E. Bride, & N. Mazza (Eds.), *Death and trauma: The traumatology of grieving* (pp. 159–192). Washington, DC: Taylor and Francis.

Session 9 When a sibling dies

Journal #4 due

Reading:

Becvar, chapter 7

Rigazio-Digilio, S. A. (2001). Videography: Re-storying the lives of clients facing terminal illness. In R. Neimeyer (Ed.), *Meaning reconstruction and the experience of loss* (pp. 331–344). Washington, DC: American Psychological Association.

Session 10 When a parent dies

Assignment #3 due

Reading:

Becvar, chapter 8

Worden, J. W. (1996). *Children and grief.* New York: Guilford Press (pp. 139–169).

Session 11 When a spouse dies

Journal #5 due

Reading:

Becvar, chapter 9

Baker, J. E. (1997). Minimizing the impact of parental grief on children: Parent and family interventions. In C. R. Figley, B. E. Bride, & N. Mazza (Eds.), *Death and trauma: The traumatology of grieving* (pp. 139–157). Washington, DC: Taylor and Francis.

Session 12 When an extended family member or friend dies

Reading:

Becvar, chapter 10

Boss, P., Beaulieu, L. Wieling, E., Turner, W., & LaCruz, S. (2003). Healing loss, ambiguity, and trauma: A community-based intervention with families of union workers missing after the 9/11 attack in New York City. *Journal of Marital and Family Therapy, 29*(4), 455–467.

Turner, W. G. (2003). Bereavement counseling: Using a social work model for pet loss. *Journal of Family Social Work, 7*(1), 69–81.

Session 13 Creating funerals, ceremonies, and other healing rituals
Journal #6 due

Reading:
Becvar, chapter 11
McGoldrick, M. (2004). Echoes from the past: Helping families deal with their ghosts. In F. Walsh & M. McGoldrick (Eds.), *Living beyond loss: Death in the family* (2nd ed., pp. 310–339). New York: Guilford Press.

Session 14 Searching for meaning / reclaiming joy

Reading:
Becvar, chapters 12 and 13
Sedney, M. A., Baker, J. E., & Gross, E. (1994). "The story" of a death: Therapeutic considerations with bereaved families. *Journal of Marital and Family Therapy, 20*(3), 287–296.
Session 15 Assignment #4 due
Final journal due

Session 16 Assignment #4 due

BIBLIOGRAPHY

Cultural Perspectives on Death and Dying

Becker, E. (1973). *The denial of death*. New York: Free Press.
Kalish, R. A. (Ed.). (1980). *Death and dying: Views from many cultures*. Farmingdale, NY: Baywood.
Kapleau, P. (1989). *The wheel of life and death*. New York: Doubleday.
Kastenbaum, R. J. (1986). *Death, society, and human experience* (3rd. ed.). Columbus, OH: Charles E. Merrill.
Mitford, J. (1963). *The American way of death*. New York: Simon and Schuster.
Mitford, J. (2000). *The American way of death revisited*. New York: Vintage Books.
Shneidman, E. S. (Ed.). (1980). *Death: Current perspectives* (2nd. ed.). Palo Alto, CA: Mayfield.
Stiller, B. C. (2001). *What happens when I die?* Colorado Springs, CO: Pinon Press.

Grief

Becvar, D. (2000). Families experiencing death, dying and bereavement. In W. C. Nichols, M. A., Nichols, D. S. Becvar, & A. Y. Napier (Eds.), *The handbook of family development and intervention* (pp. 453–470). New York: John Wiley.
Becvar, D. S. (2001). *In the presence of grief: Helping family members successfully*

resolve death, dying, bereavement and related end of life issues. New York: Guilford Press.
Berkus, R. (1984). *To heal again: Towards serenity and the resolution of grief.* Encino, CA: Red Rose Press.
Bouvard, M., & Gladu, E. (1998). *The path through grief: A compassionate guide*. New York: Prometheus Books.
Deits, B. (1988). *Life after loss: A personal guide to dealing with death, divorce, job change and relocation*. Tuscon, AZ: Fisher Books.
Figley, C. R., Bride, B. E., & Mazza, N. (Eds.). (1997). *Death and trauma: The traumatology of grieving*. Washington, DC: Taylor and Francis.
Klass, D., Silverman, P. R., & Nickman, S. (Eds.). (1996). *Continuing bonds: New understandings of grief.* Washington, DC: Taylor and Francis.
Kübler-Ross, E. (1969). *On death and dying*. New York: Macmillan.
Kübler-Ross, E. (1975). *Death: The final stage of growth*. New York: Touchstone.
Kübler-Ross, E. (1995). *Death is of vital importance*. New York: Station Hill Press.
Kübler-Ross, E. (1997). *The wheel of life and death: A memoir of living and dying*. New York: Scribner.
Kushner, H. S. (1981). *When bad things happen to good people*. New York: Avon Books.
Levang, E. (1998). *When men grieve: Why men grieve differently and how you can help*. Minneapolis, MN: Fairview Press.
Lightner, C., & Hathaway, N. (1990). *Giving sorrow words: How to cope with grief and get on with your life*. New York: Warner Books.
Nolen-Hoeksema, S., & Larson, J. (1999). *Coping with loss*. Mahwah, NY: Lawrence Erlbaum.
Osterweis, M., Solomon, F., & Green, M. (Eds.). (1984). *Bereavement: Reactions, consequences, and care*. Washington, DC: National Academy Press.
Raphael, B. (1983). *The anatomy of bereavement*. New York: Basic Books.
Shapiro, E. R. (1994). *Grief as a family process: A developmental approach to clinical practice*. New York: Guilford Press.
Strommen, M. P., & Strommen, A. I. (1993). *Five cries of grief.* New York: HarperCollins.
Walsh, F., & McGoldrick, M. (2004). *Living beyond loss: Death in the family* (2nd ed.). New York: W. W. Norton.

Loss of a Child

Bernstein, J. (1997). *When the bough breaks: Forever after the death of a son or daughter.* Kansas City, MO: Andrews and McKeel.
Bramblett, J. (1991). *When good-bye is forever: Learning to live again after the loss of a child*. New York: Ballantine Books.
Claypool, J. (1974). *Tracks of a fellow struggler: How to handle grief.* Waco, TX: Word Books.
Jurgensen, G. (1999). *The disappearance*. New York: W. W. Norton.
Klass, D. (1988). *Parental grief: Solace and resolution*. New York: Springer.
Knapp, R. (1986). *Beyond endurance: When a child dies*. New York: Shocken.
Kohner, N., & Henley, A. (1997). *When a baby dies: The experience of late miscarriage, stillbirth and neonatal death*. London: Thorsons.

McCracken, A., & Semel, M. (1998). *A broken heart still beats: After the death of a child.* Center City, MN: Hazelden.
Schiff, H. S. (1977). *The bereaved parent.* New York: Penguin.
Wolterstorff, N. (1987). *Lament for a son.* Grand Rapids, MI: William B. Eerdmans.

Loss of a Sibling

Bernstein, J. (2000). *Bereft: A sister's story.* New York: North Point Press.
Rosen, H. (1986). *Unspoken grief: Coping with childhood sibling loss.* Lexington, MA: Lexington Books.

Loss of a Parent

Brooks, J. (1999). *Midlife orphan: Facing life's changes now that your parents are gone.* New York: Berkley Books.
Edelman, H. (1994). *Motherless daughters: The legacy of loss.* New York: Dell.
Kennedy, A. (1991). *Losing a parent: Passage to a new way of living.* New York: HarperCollins

Loss of a Spouse

Lewis, C. S. (1976). *A grief observed.* New York: Seabury Press.
Van Auken, S. (1977). *A severe mercy.* San Francisco: Harper and Row.
Zonnebelt-Smeenge, S. J., & De Vries, R. C. (1998). *Getting to the other side of grief: Overcoming the loss of a spouse.* Grand Rapids, MI: Baker Books.

Loss of a Friend

Smith, H. I. (1996). *Grieving the death of a friend.* Minneapolis, MN: Augsburg Fortress.

Loss of a Pet

O'Maley, C. (2000, February 24). Pet death should be taken seriously. *Butler Collegian.*
Rosenberg, M. A. (1986). *Companion animal loss and pet owner grief.* ALPO Pet Center.

Ambiguous Loss

Boss, P. (1999). *Ambiguous loss: Learning to live with unresolved grief.* Cambridge, MA: Harvard Univesity Press.

Suicide

Hendin, H. (1995). *Suicide in America.* New York: W. W. Norton.
Shneidman, E. S. (1996). *The suicidal mind.* New York: Oxford University Press.

End-of-Life Issues

Battin, M. (1994). *The least worst death: Essays in bioethics on the end of life.* New York: Oxford University Press.

Becvar, D. (2000). Euthanasia decisions. In F. W. Kaslow (Ed.), *Handbook of couple and family forensic issues* (pp. 439–458). New York: John Wiley.

Byock, I. (1997). *Dying well.* New York: Riverhead Books.

Callanan, M., & Kelley, P. (1992). *Final gifts: Understanding the special awareness, needs, and communications of the dying.* New York: Bantam Books.

Carlson, L. (1987). *Caring for the dead: Your final act of love.* Hinesburg, VT: Upper Access.

Choice in Dying. (1991). *Refusal of treatment legislation: A state by state compilation of enacted and model statutes.* New York: Author.

Dworkin, R. (1993). *Life's dominion: An argument about abortion and euthanasia.* London: HarperCollins.

Dying Well Network. (1996). *Helping people die well.* Spokane, WA: Author.

Farberman, R. K. (1997). *Terminal illness and hastened death requests: The important role of the mental health professional.* Washington, DC: American Psychological Association.

Foos-Graber, A. (1989). *Deathing: An intelligent alternative for the final moments of life.* York Beach, ME: Nicolas-Hays.

Groopman, J. (1997). *The measure of our days: New beginnings at life's end.* New York: Viking.

Humphrey, D., & Clement, M. (2000). *People, politics and the right-to-die movement.* New York: St. Martin's Griffin.

Kramp, E. T., & Kramp, D. H. (1998). *Living with the end in mind.* New York: Three Rivers Press.

Kreilkamp, A. (1999). Caring for our own dead: Interview with Jerri Lyons. *Crone Chronicles, 41,* 20–30, 51.

Kuhl, D. (2002). *What dying people want: Practical wisdom for the end of life.* New York: Public Affairs.

Levine, S. (1982). *Who dies? An investigation of conscious living and conscious dying.* New York: Doubleday.

Levine, S. (1997). *One year to live: How to live this year as if it were your last.* New York: Bell Tower.

Madden, K. (1999). *Shamanic guide to death and dying.* St. Paul, MN: Llewellyn Publications.

Nouwen, H. J. M. (1994). *Our greatest gift: A meditation of dying and caring.* New York: HarperCollins.

Sogyal, R. (1992). *The Tibetan book of living and dying.* New York: HarperCollins.

Starhawk, N. M. M., & the Reclaiming Collective. (1997). *The pagan book of living and dying.* New York: HarperCollins.

Life after Life

Anderson, G., & Barone, A. (2000). *George Anderson's lessons from the light: Extraordinary messages of comfort and hope from the other side.* New York: Berkley Books.

Coddington, R. H. (1987). *Death brings many surprises.* New York: Ivy Books.
Martin, J., & Romanowski, P. (1994). *Our children forever: Messages from children on the other side.* New York: Berkley Books.
Moody, R. A. (1977). *Life after life: The investigation of a phenomenom—survival of bodily death.* New York: Bantam.
Morse, M. (1990). *Closer to the light: Learning from the near-death experiences of children.* New York: Ivy Books.
Ring, K. (1984). *Heading toward omega: In search of the meaning of the near-death experience.* New York: William Morrow.
Rothschild, J. (2000). *Signals: An inspiring story of life after life.* Novato, CA: New World Library.
Sherman, H. (1981). *The dead are alive: They can and do communicate with you.* New York: Fawcett Gold Medal.
Steiner, R. (1968). *Life between death and rebirth.* Spring Valley, NY: Anthroposophic Press.
Van Praagh, J. (2000). *Healing grief: Reclaiming life after any loss.* New York: Penguin Putnam.
Whitton, J. L., & Fisher, J. (1986). *Life between life.* New York: Warner Books.

Children's Books

Bereaved Parents of the USA–St. Louis Chapter. (n.d.). *Taste of heaven.* St. Louis, MO: Author.
Berkus, R. (2002). *To heal again: Toward serenity and the resolution of grief.* Los Angeles, CA: Red Rose Press.
Blackburn, L. B. (1987). *Timothy Duck: The story of the death of a friend.* Omaha, NE: Centering Corporation.
Blume, J. (1981). *Tiger eyes.* New York: Bantam Doubleday Dell Books for Young Readers.
Brown, M. W. (1985). *The dead bird.* New York: Harper and Row.
Buchanan-Smith, D., & Wimmer, W. (2004). *A taste of blackberries.* New York: HarperCollins.
Buscaglia, L. (1982). *The fall of Freddie the leaf.* Thorofare, NJ: Slack.
Carrick, C., & Carrick, D. (1984). *The accident.* Boston: Houghton-Mifflin.
Coerr, E. (1999). *Sadako and the thousand paper cranes.* New York: Puffin.
Companion Arts. (n.d.) *Graceful passages: A companion for living and dying.* Novato, CA: Author.
DePaula, T. (2000). *Nana upstairs and Nana downstairs.* New York: Putnam Juvenile.
Dragonwagon, C. (1990). *Winter holding spring.* New York: Atheneum Books for Young Readers.
Fassier, J. (1983). *My grandpa died today.* Marshalls Creek, PA: Shawnee Press.
Gregory, V. (1992). *Through the mickle woods.* Boston: Little, Brown.
Grollman, E. A. (1991). *Talking about death: A dialogue between parent and child.* Boston: Beacon Press.
Hanson, W. (1997). *The next place.* Minneapolis, MN: Waldman House.
Hazen, B. S. (1985). *Why did Grandpa die?* New York: Golden Book.

Heegaard, M. (1988). *When someone very special dies.* Minneapolis, MN: Woodland Press.
Hughes, P. (1978). *Dying is different.* Mahomet, IL: Mech Mentor Educational Publishers.
Krebs, P. (1982). *It's hard to tell you how I feel.* Minneapolis, MN: Augsburg Fortress.
Krementz, J. (1988). *How it feels when a parent dies.* New York: Knopf.
Kübler-Ross, E. (1982). *Remember the secret.* Berkeley, CA: Celestial Arts
LeTour, K. (1987). *For those who live: Helping children cope with the death of a brother or sister.* Omaha, NE: Centering Corporation.
Lionni, L. (1967). *Frederick.* New York: Knopf.
Lopez, B. (1990). *Crow and weasel.* San Francisco: North Point Press.
Mann, P. (1979). *There are two kinds of terrible.* Minneapolis, MN: Avon Books.
Mellonie, B., & Ingpen, R. (1989). *Beginnings and endings with lifetimes in between.* Penguin Books Australia.
Paulus, T. (1972). *Hope for the flowers.* New York: Paulist Press.
Schwiebert, P., & DeKlyen, C. (1999). *Tear soup.* Portland, OR: Grief Watch.
Scribani, M. (1987). *Love, Mark.* Syracuse, NY: Hope for Bereaved.
Seuss, Dr. (1986). *You're only old once.* New York: Random House.
Shles, L. M. (1983). *Moths and fathers, feathers and mothers.* St. Louis, MO: Squib.
Shles, L. M. (1985). *Hoots and toots and hairy brutes.* Boston: Houghton Mifflin.
Stein, S. B. (1983). *About dying.* New York: Walker.
Stickney, D. (1982). *Water bugs and dragon-flies.* New York: Pilgrim Press.
Sullivan, E. (1969). *Walter Fish.* Canfield, OH: Alba House Communications.
Viorst, J. (1971). *The tenth good thing about Barney.* New York: Aladdin.
Walker, A. (1988). *To hell with dying.* San Diego, CA: Harcourt Brace Jovanovich.
Willliams, M. (1975). *The velveteen rabbit.*New York: Avon Books.

Perspectives on Dying Personal Questionnaire

1. My first personal involvement with death was with:
   a. a grandparent or great-grandparent
   b. a parent
   c. a brother or sister
   d. a other family member
   e. a friend or acquaintance
   f. a stranger
   g. a public figure
   h. a pet
2. What was your reaction to the above event, and how did others around you respond?
3. When I was young, the subject of dying was talked about in my family:
   a. openly
   b with some sense of discomfort
   c. only when necessary and then with an attempt to exclude me
   d. as though it were a taboo subject
   e. I never recall any discussion.
4. My childhood concept of what happens after death is best described as:
   a. heaven and hell
   b. afterlife
   c. asleep
   d. cessation of all physical and mental activity
   e. mysterious and unknowable
   f. something other than the above
   g. no concept
   h. can't remember
5. Today, my concept of what happens after death is:
6. My present attitudes toward dying have been most influenced by:
   a. the death of someone close
   b. specific reading
   c. religious upbringing
   d. introspection and meditation
   e. ritual (e.g., funerals)

f. TV, radio, or motion pictures
g. longevity of my family
h. my health or a physical condition
i. other people
j. other (please describe)

7. The role that religion has played in the development of my attitudes about dying is:

a. very important
b. rather important
c. minor
d. none at all

8. I think about dying:

a. very frequently (at least once a day)
b. frequently
c. occasionally
d. rarely (no more than once a year)
e. very rarely or never

9. To me, death means:

a. the end—the final process of life
b. beginning of a life after death
c. a joining of the spirit with a universal cosmic consciousness
d. a kind of endless sleep; rest; peace
e. termination of this life but with survival of the spirit
f. don't know

10. The following statement describes the degree of effort that I feel should be made to keep a terminally ill person alive:

a. All possible effort should be made.
b. Efforts that are reasonable for the person's age, physical condition, mental condition, and pain should be made.
c. After reasonable care has been given, a person ought to be permitted to die a natural death.
d. A person should not be kept alive by elaborate artificial means.

11. When I think of dying or when I become aware of my own mortality, I feel:

a. fearful
b. discouraged
c. depressed
d. purposeless
e. resolved in relation to life

f. pleasure in being alive
g. other reactions (please describe)

12. How much thought have you given to your own death in terms of when and how you might die or might prefer to die?
    a. none at all
    b. some
    c. a great deal

Personal Timeline

Starting with the year that you were born, chart the major events or milestones in your life up to the present time. Indicate the event, the year, and your age at the time. You may mark a number on the line and provide a key to the numbers below if you desire:

Birth Present

Thinking about Your Life, Your Dying, and Your Death

1. Situate yourself on the following lifeline in terms of how long you have lived since birth and how much time you believe you have left until your death:

Birth ____ Death

2. What percentage of your life have you already lived?
3. How much time do you believe you have left?
4. How do you think you will die?
5. How would you prefer to die?
6. Have you made a living will?
7. Do you intend to donate any part of your body?
8. What kind of after-death wishes do you have for disposal of your body?
9. What kind of funeral or other ceremony would you like?
10. Do you like the way you have spent your time so far?
11. Do you believe you have been here before?
12. Do you believe you will be here again?
13. Where do you believe you have come from?
14. Where do you believe you will go when you die?
15. What is the meaning of time for you?
16. Are you on the road going somewhere?
17. Do you want to be going there?
18. Do you have a life mission?
19. Is where you are right now all right with you?
20. Write your obituary as well as an epitaph for your gravestone. Write for the time in the future when you anticipate you will die, and take into consideration what you will have accomplished by then and how your death occurs.

LIFE EVENTS INVENTORY

Certain life events can result in major changes in a person's life. Death of a family member or loved one, marriage, relationship issues, changes in circumstances and conditions of employment, illness, and injury are examples of major life events. Such life events usually result in deep emotional shifts. They compromise your attention and energy and can dispose you to injury or illness. Consequently, they can adversely affect your ability to cope with the demands of daily living.

Apparently, even positive life events carry the same risk of illness and injury as those that weaken or harm us. Life events are unavoidable, and they tend to affect our ability to cope. The purpose of this inventory is to give you a tool to measure the events in your life that affect your ability to cope. In doing so, you will be prepared to identify the source of any distress and seek appropriate remediation, including health care and self-care.

This inventory was designed to be administered at least once a year. Of course, it can be administered more often if you wish. Use it to measure how well you are doing and what influences are at play in your life.

There is nothing magical about the Life Events Inventory or any other worksheet—they are simply self-assessment and problem-solving tools. They are very helpful since they can be used to track and measure your impairments as well as your improvements. They can help you prepare for medical appointments by identifying problems or patterns that you wish to discuss with your doctor. Additionally, they can be used to track things that are not especially problematic but represent things that you may want to change in yourself.

Instructions: The following pages contain a list of events that might bring about changes in a person's life. Think about the past twelve months of your life, and check off "yes" if the event occurred in your life in the past twelve months, and "no" if it did not. In the blank space next to each item, describe how you are coping with that particular item (e.g., relying on friends, family members, doctors, spiritual leader, medication; figuring out who to blame; still mourning; working through it or over it; celebrating).

Adapted from National Institutes of Health. (1998, October). *Traumatic brain injury rehabilitation consensus statement.* Available at http://www.headinjury.com/lifevents.htm

Life event in the past twelve months	Yes	No	Describe how you are coping
1. Became disabled or incapacitated			
2. Loss of sense of self			
3. Loss of independence			
4. Loss of identity and stature			
5. Became dependent on others for basic subsistence			
6. Became dependent on others for personal care and maintenance			
7. Loss of self-determination and self-sufficiency			
8. Loss of personal mobility			
9. Loss of previous capacities and capabilities			
10. Sexual problems			
11. Experienced infidelity			
12. Divorce or separation			
13. Change in closeness with spouse, lover, partner			
14. Reconciled with spouse, lover, partner			
15. Ongoing conflict with present spouse, lover, partner			
16. Conflict with parents, siblings, family members			
17. Problems with former spouse, lover, partner			
18. Social isolation			
19. Change in social activities			
20. Family turmoil			
21. Became engaged			
22. Married or began a live-in relationship			
23. Problems with co-workers			
24. Work interfered with family life			
25. You or partner fired			
26. Major change in conditions of work			
27. Death of a spouse, lover, or other family member			

Life event in the past twelve months	Yes	No	Describe how you are coping
28. Death of a child (including miscarriage or stillbirth)			
29. Pregnancy			
30. Became a parent			
31. Child or family member left home			
32. Child returned home with a child, etc.			
33. Change in marital status of your children or parents			
34. Gained new live-in family member			
35. Changed residence			
36. Landlord problems			
37. Mortgage or loan foreclosure			
38. Became homeless			
39. Moved to new town			
40. Loss of regular transportation			
41. Began adolescence			
42. Graduated from high school or college			
43. Embarked on new career			
44. Began menopause			
45. Other major life change			
46. Long-term or life-threatening illness or injury			
47. Major change in health or behavior of family or friend			
48. Long-term illness, injury, or disability of household member			
49. Death of family or household member			
50. Made a major decision regarding your immediate future			
51. Major personal achievement.			
52. Change in your personal habits, lifestyle, dress, hobbies			
53. Change in your religious or political beliefs			
54. Loss or damage to personal property			

Life event in the past twelve months	Yes	No	Describe how you are coping
55. Vacation			
56. Trip, not a vacation			
57. Christmas/Thanksgiving, or other major holiday			
58. Change in family get-togethers			
59. Change in your social activities			
60. Made a new friend			
61. Broke up with a friend due to conflict			
62. Lost friend for any other reason (e.g., death, moving)			
63. Major change in finances			
64. New purchase (e.g., car)			
65. New mortgage loan			
66. Credit rating difficulties			
67. Victim of a violent crime			
68. Physical abuse by partner, parent, caregiver, other			
69. Emotional abuse			
70. Injured in car or other accident			
71. Involved in injury claim or lawsuit			
72. Lawsuit against you			
73. Jailed due to legal trouble			
74. Victim of natural disaster			
75. Change in sleep habits			
76. Change in diet and appetite			
77. Developed thinking and learning disabilities			
78. Developed problems with emotional control			
79. Sudden decline in grades			
80. Asked to withdraw from school, or dropped out of school			
81. Conflict with school officials			
82. Conflict with classmates			
83. Change in child care			
84. Parenting conflicts			
85. Conflicts with children			

Life event in the past twelve months	Yes	No	Describe how you are coping
86. Single parenting			
87. Custody battles			
88. Child abuse issues.			
89. Learning-disabled child			
90. Emotionally fragile child			
Total “yes” responses			

24

Social Work Practice with Grief and Loss

Mark de St. Aubin

COURSE DESCRIPTION

This course presents models of grief and bereavement that will be applied in practice with individuals. Emphasis will be placed on the direct practice knowledge and clinical skills understood in the profession to constitute what is called grief therapy.

In addition to the experience of losing a significant other as a result of death, grief/bereavement from other losses (e.g., functional level, role, independence, meaning, hopes) will also be considered across the life span. Psychodynamic (Bowlby), stage (Kübler-Ross), and task theories (Worden) of grief will be applied to the process of mourning and will be used to guide students in their development of clinical skills with this population. Diverse cultural and faith perspectives will be examined in readings and class discussion. The challenges of mourning specific losses and the practice methods necessary to facilitate the healthy grieving of these will also be discussed.

The student will be required to explore his or her own loss history and grief experiences, both in quiet introspection and in class. This personal grief work is believed to be essential to one's own effectiveness as a grief therapist since one cannot accompany a client into territory that one has not traveled.

COURSE OBJECTIVES

At the conclusion of the course, students will be able to:

- Appreciate the impact of culture and religious beliefs on clients and their families in relation to their process of bereavement and mourning
- Commit to the principle that regardless of culture, ethnicity, sexual orientation, gender, lifestyle, or socioeconomic status, each individual has great worth and should be treated with respect
- Demonstrate an understanding of each client's right to self-determination in his or her expression of grief and grief rituals

- Understand the impact of various losses on individuals and their families
- Demonstrate knowledge of several accepted theories of grief and mourning and apply these to a variety of populations
- Demonstrate knowledge of the four tasks of mourning and the barriers to their achievement
- Articulate common individual and family responses to loss, both adaptive and maladaptive
- Demonstrate knowledge of specific clinical interventions that can facilitate grief resolution (for both complicated and uncomplicated grief)
- Demonstrate mastery of the foundation skills of client engagement
- Support a client's present state and expression of grief through verbal and behavioral skills that allow the client to grieve in his or her own way
- Demonstrate moderate proficiency of clinical interventions in facilitating a client's accomplishment of each of the four tasks of mourning

TEXTS

Viorst, J. (1986). *Necessary losses*. New York: Simon and Schuster.
Worden, J. W. (1991). *Grief counseling and grief therapy: A handbook for the mental health practitioner* (2nd ed.). New York: Springer.

ASSIGNMENTS

Personal Journal: Each student will keep a personal journal of thoughts and emotions that come up for him or her each week as a result of the readings and class discussion. Each week's journal entry will be turned in at the start of each class period and will be graded credit/no credit.

Quizzes: There will be a total of ten quizzes throughout the term. These quizzes will be given weekly at the beginning of class. Students will be allowed to drop their lowest quiz grade before final grades are computed.

Videotaped Sessions: Each student will be responsible for creating a video excerpt of client work (or work with another individual in role play). This video takes the place of the final exam. By the time class is winding up, each student should have learned how to apply and use most of the principles of grief therapy at a beginning or intermediate level of proficiency. To demonstrate what he or she has learned, the student will videotape a complete twenty-minute session with a patient/client from his or her agency (or with another student role-playing as a patient/client), using interventions addressing each of the four tasks of mourning discussed in class. This tape will then be reviewed with the instructor. In addition to the videotaped session, the student will turn in a process recording of the session that analyzes the student/therapist work with the patient/client. The instructor will not be critical of "mistakes" made by the student during the session but, rather, will look for the student's examination of his or her own understanding of the course content as this relates to the patient/client interaction during the session. The majority of the grade for this assignment will be based on the content of the process and the student's critical analysis of his or her own session.

COURSE OUTLINE

Session 1 Introductions and course overview
Personal relationship to grief/loss
Grief theories
Review of foundation skills of client engagement

Session 2 Introduction to Worden model: Four tasks of mourning
Hand in journal entry
Quiz #1
Reading: Worden, chapters 1 and 2
Discussion
Clinical practice

Session 3 Grief counseling
Facilitating uncomplicated grief
Hand in journal entry
Quiz #2
Reading: Worden, chapter 3
Discussion
Clinical practice

Session 4 Losses throughout the life span (part 1)
Hand in journal entry
Quiz #3
Reading: Viorst, chapters 1–10
Discussion
Clinical practice

Session 5 Losses throughout the life span (part 2)
Hand in journal entry
Quiz #4
Reading: Viorst, chapters 11–20

Session 6	Abnormal grief reactions: Complicated mourning Resolving pathological grief Hand in journal entry Quiz #5 Reading: Worden, chapters 4 and 5 Discussion Clinical practice
Session 7	Grieving special types of losses Suicide, sudden death, AIDS, murder, and conflictual relationships Hand in journal entry Quiz #6 Reading: Worden, chapter 6 Discussion Clinical practice
Session 8	Grieving special types of losses Parents who lose a child, SIDS, miscarriages, abortions Hand in journal entry Quiz #7 Reading: Worden, chapter 6 Discussion Clinical practice
Session 9	Children's grief and mourning Field trip Hand in journal entry Quiz #8 Reading: TBA Discussion
Session 10	Care of the dead body: A visit to a funeral home Hand in journal entry No readings Discussion
Session 11	Use of ritual in facilitating grief Guest speaker Hand in journal entry Quiz #9 Reading: TBA Discussion Clinical practice
Session 12	Working with the dying: Anticipatory grief Hand in journal entry

	Quiz #10 Reading: TBA Discussion Clinical practice
Session 13	Diversity and grief: Panel of religious and cultural representatives Hand in journal entry No readings Discussion
Session 14	Current research in bereavement studies Guest speaker from gerontology center Hand in journal entry No reading Discussion Clinical practice

25

Loss and Grief

Individual, Family, and Cultural Perspectives

Diane Green

"The world is full of suffering; it is also full of overcoming suffering."
—Helen Keller

COURSE DESCRIPTION

This course will give students an opportunity to explore their perceptions and beliefs about death and dying and how individual cultural differences influence that experience and prepare them for working with clients on grief and loss. The course examines issues of death and dying, grief processes, and sense of meaning, including coping and adaptation for individuals and families as they deal with various kinds of loss. We will look at a range of factors (involving the individual, family, community, and society) that can affect, impede, or facilitate the grief experiences of individuals and families. Grief will be explored from a life-span developmental perspective (from prenatal development through late adulthood) within the context of varied types of family and sociocultural systems. An emphasis will be placed on both personal and professional applications of course information.

The philosophy underlying this course is in line with the "Statements on Death, Dying and Bereavement" (1994) of the International Work Group on Death, Dying, and Bereavement. The introduction states: "Death, dying, and bereavement are fundamental and pervasive aspects of the human experience. Individuals and societies can only achieve fullness of living by understanding and appreciating these realities. The absence of such understanding and appreciation may result in unnecessary suffering, loss of dignity, alienation, and diminished quality of living. Therefore, education about death, dying, and bereavement is an essential component of the educational process at all levels, both formal and informal."

For additional documents developed by the International Work Group on Death, Dying, and Bereavement, check out their Web site at http://maxwell.psyc.memphis.edu/iwg.

COURSE GOALS

This course strives to examine issues of grief and loss as they are experienced across the life span of the individual, within family contexts, and across families' histories. Families are seen as systems in which relationships are influenced by meanings derived from actions and interactions, communication, beliefs, and expectations. Family, individual, and sociocultural factors combine to affect grief and its place in our lives. Grief can occur in relation to many types of losses, including physical or psychological absence, as well as the loss of dreams and meaning. In this course we will view experiences of loss, such as deaths, as having the potential to concurrently produce change, deterioration, and growth.

By the end of this course, students should be able to:

- Define and contrast the meanings and applications of bereavement, grief, and mourning
- Identify their own loss histories and beliefs and differentiate their personal boundaries from their professional roles
- Comprehend the developmental impact of bereavement, grief, and mourning within the life span of an individual and the family
- Explore the various determinants of grief and their impact on the tasks of mourning
- Facilitate discussion of diverse cultural, geographical, spiritual, ethnic, and psychosocial factors related to grief, loss, and mourning
- Apply a health perspective in assessments and clinical interventions
- Recognize the emotional, behavioral, cognitive, physical, and spiritual expressions that accompany bereavement, grief, and mourning
- Identify various community referral networks for loss-specific services
- Define compassion fatigue and explore patterns for self-care in a work environment of multiple loss and grief
- Critically analyze material related to the course subject
- Critically analyze and assess values and ethical dilemmas regarding death, dying, grief, and loss (such as end-of-life decision making)
- Demonstrate strategies designed to reduce discrimination and oppression regarding death-and-dying issues and explore the various determinants of grief and their impact on the tasks of mourning with various at-risk populations

- Examine and critically evaluate various community referral networks for loss-specific services and policy implications of end-of-life decision making
- Demonstrate practice competence in grief-and-loss issues within an ecological framework

This is an advanced curriculum course that builds on both the human behavior courses and the practice courses taught in the foundation curriculum. It is assumed that the student is acquainted with the impact of general stress on individuals, families, and communities and is familiar with a variety of social work practice methods considered effective in work with these populations. Grief affects people of all ages and cultures; it is found in clients in most settings. Therefore, the work of this course is appropriate for direct service practitioners in any service and for those who plan and direct services at an agency or community level.

The practice skills students may anticipate developing as a result of completing this course are:

- The ability to conduct a grief assessment based on the particular characteristics of a loss due to death
- The ability to apply the health perspective in developing a plan of care for grieving clients
- The ability to plan and implement a bereavement support group
- The ability to use the processes of grief to intervene clinically with individuals and families
- The ability to make effective referrals for loss-specific services

TEACHING METHODS

The teaching format will consist of experiential exercises, lectures, discussions, and audiovisual media to help students understand and integrate their own beliefs of death and dying into their social work practice. Throughout the course, students will be asked to focus on cultural influences, including gender, age, sexual orientation, spiritual beliefs, socioeconomic, and language differences, as well as individuals with developmental disabilities. Ethics and values associated with the dying process and death-and-grief reactions will also be examined throughout the course with a variety of populations.

REQUIRED TEXTS

Corr, C. A., Nabe, C. M., & Corr, D. M. (2003). *Death and dying: Life and living*. Belmont, CA: Wadsworth/Thomson Learning.

Irish, D. P., Lundquist, K. F., & Nelson, V. J. (Eds.). (1993). *Ethnic variations in dying, death and grief: Diversity in universality.* Washington, DC: Taylor and Francis.
Neimeyer, R. (2001). *Meaning and reconstruction and the experience of loss.* Washington, DC: American Psychological Association

COURSE ASSIGNMENTS AND GRADING

Attendance and class participation are critical factors in the learning process for this course. It is expected that students will complete readings and assignments prior to class and will come prepared to contribute to class discussions.

Book/film critique	20%
Grief interview	25%
Field trip	15%
Cultural presentation	20%
Logs	10%
Class participation/attendance	10%
Total	100%

Critique of a film or book: Students are required to write one critique (3–5 pages in length) discussing the issues of death and dying as portrayed in either a film or a book (your choice). Film or book reviews are not acceptable. Students are expected to apply their knowledge, experience, and personal thoughts regarding grief and loss to examine the story and compare and contrast their own perceptions of the grief issues and how they were handled. Critiques will be discussed in class after papers are turned in. See below for suggested books and films for this assignment. Other films and books may be used with the permission of the instructor.

In *You Can Go Home Again,* Monica McGoldrick states: "Questions are the most powerful tool for gaining a new understanding of losses." The questions below may be used as a guide for subject points in writing the critiques, but it is expected that students' approach will be comprehensive. Critiques should address—but not be limited to—the following questions.

- How did various family members express their reactions to death? Did they talk to one another about the death?
- Who was present at the moment of death? Who was not present, and who should have been?
- How were family relationships at the time of death? Did any family members have unresolved issues with the person who died?
- Who arranged the funeral? Who attended? Who didn't? Who gave the eulogy?

- Was the body cremated or buried? If it was cremated, what happened to the ashes? Is there a marking of the grave?
- Did family conflicts or cutoffs occur around the time of death?
- Was there a will? Who received what bequests? Were there family rifts because of provisions in the will?
- Do family members visit the grave, and if so, how often? Who mentions the dead person, and with what frequency? What happened to the belongings of the dead person?
- Is there secrecy about the cause or circumstance of the death? Were facts kept from anyone inside or outside the family?
- What mythology has been created in the family about the dead person? Has he or she been idealized?
- What would the history of the family have been like if the dead person had survived longer?
- Do family members feel stigmatized by the death (e.g,. suicide, a death from AIDS)?
- How have the survivors' lives been influenced by their relationships with the deceased? What do they carry with them from him or her?
- What are the family beliefs about afterlife, and how have these beliefs influenced the family's understanding of the meaning of loss?
- What other beliefs do family members have that may help sustain them in the face of loss (e.g., sense of family or cultural mission, a sense of survivorship)?

Grief interview (written report and class presentation): Each student is expected to submit a written report of a grief interview and present a summary of the interview. The student is expected to conduct a face-to-face interview with another individual regarding issues related to a traumatic, ambiguous, or stigmatized loss and issues related to the individual's experience of grief and depression, anxiety, or any other emotional ramifications of the loss. If the loss is a death, the death cannot have occurred within the last year. The person interviewed may be a member of the student's family if the student has enough objectivity to complete the assignment appropriately. Students are expected to use one or a combination of the structured interview questions found in assessment articles. The report (5–7 double-spaced pages, no bibliography) should be printed and turned in on the date of the class presentation. It should consist of the following sections:

Guided storytelling: This section should discuss the circumstances of the death and the impact of the death on the survivor's life (listen for secondary and symbolic losses as well as changes in the survivor's assumptive world as a result of the death); things that were done and said that were particularly helpful; support services that were used to help survivor work through his or her grief, and inner resources (including the use of rituals) that have helped with survival.

Clinical learning and personal insights: The second section should address the student's learning and how it will influence future practice and knowledge gained about personal reactions and the impact of grief.

The class presentation should be a brief summary (5–7 minutes) of the loss; however, the primary focus should be on the clinical and personal learning.

Field trip (written report): Each student is expected to visit a funeral home, cemetery, crematorium, or hospice (field placements may not be used) during the semester. Students are expected to arrange the visit on their own and write a summary of their experience. As students prepare for the field trip, they are expected to be aware of and utilize their own experiences and beliefs about death, dying, and loss. This paper should be two to three pages long.

Class presentation on diversity in religious/cultural views of death, dying, and grief: Small groups of students will work together to review the beliefs and practices of a specific religious/cultural group that relate to illness, suffering, death, dying, grief, mourning rituals, and burial. If possible, you should interview an individual of that faith or culture. If you choose a formal religion, interviewing a clergy person of that faith might be helpful. It is obvious that not every person of a particular religion or culture grieves in the same way as every other person within that group, but common themes or traditions or activities should be noted. Information on the background of the population, implications for grieving patterns, and strengths of the population for resiliency and healing in grief should be included. All members of the group will participate in making a presentation on their findings and in creating a handout and bibliography to provide to the class. Presentations should be forty-five to sixty minutes in length.

Logs: Periodically throughout the semester, students will be asked to write in a log at the end of a lecture. The logs are to be a diary in which students report and analyze their thoughts, feelings, and experiences related to the topic of the lecture. The course activities are designed to facilitate and stimulate introspection abut death, dying, and grief, and the logs should reflect that thinking. Students' ability to reflect and write about their own losses and feelings plays a crucial role in their ability to help clients with their losses. Whatever obstacles we encounter in our own grief throughout our lives become obstacles in grief work with others. In order to remain responsible and ethical professionals, we must be aware of our own ongoing struggles and vulnerabilities to loss and be able to identify and separate them from the struggles our clients experience.

COURSE OUTLINE

Session 1 Introduction
Overview of syllabus
Personal feelings about loss and grief
Grief experience inventory / self-assessment
Learning about death, dying, and bereavement
Education and death and dying
Changing encounters with death
Begin work on cultural presentation
Reading: Corr, Nabe, & Corr, chapters 1 and 2

Session 2 Death
Changing attitudes toward death
Death-related practices and the American death system
Guest speaker from hospice
Work on cultural presentation
Reading: Corr, Nabe, & Corr, chapters 3 and 4

Session 3 Dying
Coping with dying: How individuals can help
Coping with dying: How communities can help
Cultural presentation 1
Reading: Corr, Nabe, & Corr, chapters 6, 7, and 8

Session 4 Bereavement
Coping with loss and grief: How individuals can help
Coping with loss and grief: How communities can help
When a pet dies
Cultural presentation 2
Reading: Corr, Nabe, & Corr, chapters 9, 10, and 11

Session 5 Developmental perspectives
Children
Adolescents
Guest speaker from center for grieving children
Cultural presentation 3
Reading: Corr, Nabe, & Corr, chapters 12 and 13

Session 6 Developmental perspectives
Adults
Elderly
Guest speaker or film (dealing with murder, sudden death, national disasters, or tragedies and multiple deaths)
Cultural presenation 4
Reading: Corr, Nabe, & Corr, chapters 14 and 15

Session 7	Legal, conceptual, and moral issues Suicide and life-threatening behavior Assisted suicide and euthanasia: Intentionally ending a human life The meaning and place of death in life Film: *On Our Own Terms* (Moyers) Cultural presentation 5 Film/book critique due Reading: Corr, Nabe, & Corr, chapters 17, 18, and 19
Session 8	Legal, conceptual, and moral issues Legal issues Grief and HIV and AIDS Guest speaker from AIDS agency Grief interview and discussion due Reading: Corr, Nabe, & Corr, chapters 16 and 20
Session 9	Breaking ground: Toward a fresh theory of grieving Guest speaker: A child survivor of the Holocaust Cultural presentation 6 Reading: Neimeyer, chapters 1, 2, and 3
Session 10	Online class
Session 11	Reestablishing relationships: Context and connection Guest speaker from the state bar association Cultural presentation 7 Reading: Neimeyer, chapters 4, 5, and 6
Session 12	Transcending trauma: Growth after loss Cultural presentation 8 Reading: Neimeyer, chapters 7, 8, 9, and 10
Session 13	Healing stories: Research and reflexivity Cultural presentations 9 and 10 Reading: Neimeyer, chapters 11, 12, and 13
Session 14	Renegotiating the world: Making meaning in grief therapy Compassion fatigue and self-care Course closure Reading: Neimeyer, chapters 14, 15, 16, and 17
Session 15	Field trip report due Logs due

LIST OF FILMS

Philadelphia
The Color Purple
Ordinary People
Boys on the Side
Dead Poets Society
Dying Young
Forest Gump
Ghost
The Ryan White Story
Terms of Endearment
Joy Luck Club
One True Thing
Steel Magnolias
Map of the World
Sophie's Choice
Tuesdays with Morrie
A Beautiful Mind

LIST OF BOOKS

Back Roads
One True Thing
I Know This Much Is True
Map of the World
Tuesdays with Morrie
A Beautiful Mind

BIBLIOGRAPHY

For Adults/Professionals

Agee, J. (1957). *A death in the family*. New York: Grosset and Dunlap.

Akner, L. (1993). *How to survive the loss of a parent: A guide for adults*. New York: William Morrow.

Ashe, A., & Rampersad, A. (1993). *Days of grace*. New York: Ballentine Books.

Attig, T. (1996). *How we grieve: Relearning the world*. New York: Oxford University Press.

Becker, D. (1973). *The denial of death*. New York: Free Press.

Buckman, R. (1988). *I don't know what to say: How to help and support someone who is dying*. New York: Vintage Books.

Cook, A. S., & Oltjenbruns, K. A. (1998). *Dying and grieving: Life span and family perspectives*. Fort Worth, TX: Harcourt Brace.

Corless, I. B., Germino, B. B., & Pitman, M. A. (1994). *Dying, death, and bereavement: Theoretical perspectives and other ways of knowing*. Boston: Jones and Barlett.

Crenshaw, D. H. (1990). *Bereavement: Counseling the grieving throughout the life cycle*. New York: Continuum.

Edelman, H. (1994). *Motherless daughters: The legacy of loss*. New York: Dell.

Edgerton, C. (1992). *In memory of Junior.* Chapel Hill, NC: Algonquin Press.

Feinberg, L. (1994). *I'm grieving as fast as I can: How young widows and widowers can cope and heal*. Far Hills, NJ: New Horizon Press.

Fine, C. (1997). *No time to say goodbye: Surviving the suicide of a loved one*. New York: Doubleday.

Froman, P. K. (1992). *After you say goodbye: When someone you love dies of AIDS*. San Francisco: Chronicle Books.

Fulton, R., & Bendiksen, R. (1994). *Death and identity* (3rd ed.). Philadelphia: Charles Press.

Furman, D. (1974). *A child's parent dies: Studies in childhood bereavement*. New Haven, CT: Yale University Press.

Gunter, J. (1949). *Death be not proud: A memoir.* New York: Harper and Row.

Harris, M. (1996). *The loss that lasts forever.* New York: Plume.

Hennezel, M. (1997). *Intimate death: How the dying teach us how to live*. New York: Knopf.

James, J., & Cherry, F. (1988). *The grief recovery handbook: A step-by-step program for moving beyond loss*. New York: Harper and Row.

Janoff-Bulman, R. (1992). *Shattered assumptions*. New York: Free Press.

Jones, C. (1997). *R.I.P.: The complete book of death and dying*. New York: Harper-Collins.

Kennedy, A. (1991). *Losing a parent*. San Francisco: Harper.

Klass, D., Silverman, P., & Nickman, S. (Eds.). (1996). *Continuing bonds: New understandings of grief.* Washington, DC: Taylor and Francis.

Lord, J. H. (1991). *No time for goodbyes* (4th ed.). Ventura, CA: Pathfinding Publishing of California.

Lynch, T. (1997). *The undertaking: Life studies from the dismal trade*. New York: W. W. Norton.

McCourt, F. (1996). *Angela's ashes*. New York: Simon and Schuster.

McCracken, A., & Semel, M. (Eds.). (1998). *A broken heart still beats*. Center City, NJ: Hazeldon.

Mehren, E. (1997). *After the darkest hour, the sun will shine again: A parent's guide to coping with the loss of a child*. New York: Simon and Schuster.

Menton, T. (1991). *Gentle closings*. Philadelphia: Running Press.

Miller, S. (1997). *After death: Mapping the journey*. New York: Simon and Schuster.

Myers, E. (1986). *When parents die: A guide for adults*. New York: Penguin.

Publicover, R. J. L. (1993). *My unicorn has gone away: Life, death, grief, and living in the years of AIDS*. Somerville, MA: Powder House.

Rando, T. (1984). *Grief, dying, and death: Clinical interventions for caregivers*. Champaign, IL: Research Press.

Rando, T. (1991). *How to go on living when someone you love dies.* New York: Bantam Books.
Rando, T. (1999). *Clinical dimensions of anticipatory mourning: Theory and practice in working with the dying, their loved ones, and caregivers.* Champaign, IL: Research Press.
Raphael, B. (1983). *The anatomy of bereavement.* New York: Basic Books.
Redmond, L. M. (1989). *Surviving when someone you love was murdered.* Clearwater, FL: Psychological Consultation and Education Services.
Rubin, T. I. (1969). *The angry book.* Toronto: Collier Books.
Sprang, G., & McNeil, J. (1995). *The many faces of bereavement.* New York: Brunner/Mazel.
Spungen, D. (1998). *Homicide: The hidden victims.* Thousand Oaks, CA: Sage.
Straudacher, C. (1971). *Men and grief.* Oakland, CA: New Harbinger.
Twain, M. (1959). *The autobiography of Mark Twain.* New York: Harper and Row.
Viorst, J. (1986). *Necessary losses.* New York: Fawcett Columbine.
Wilber, K. (1991). *Grace and grit: Spirituality and healing in the life and death of Treya Killam Wilber.* Boston: Shambhala Publications.
Wolfelt, A. D. (1992). *Understanding grief: Helping yourself heal.* Bristol, PA: Accelerated Development.
Worden, W. (1991). *Grief counseling and grief therapy: A handbook for the mental health practitioner* (2nd ed.). New York: Springer.

Theological

Beuchner, F. (1991). *Telling secrets.* San Francisco: Harper and Row.
Claypool, J. R. (1974). *Tracks of a fellow struggler.* Waco, TX: Word Books.
Flanigan, B. (1992). *Forgiving the unforgivable.* Old Tappan, NJ: Macmillan.
Johnson, L. D. (1978). *The morning after death.* Nashville, TN: Broadman.
Lewis, C. S. (1961). *A grief observed.* New York: Seabury.
Magida, A. (Ed.). (1996). *How to be a perfect stranger.* Woodstock, VT: Jewish Lights.
Weatherhead, L. D. (1944). *The will of God.* Nashville, TN: Abingdon.
Wolterstorff, N. (1987). *Lament for a son.* Grand Rapids: MI: William B. Eerdmans.

For Teens

Buscaglia, L. (1982). *The fall of Freddie the leaf.* Thorofare, NJ: Slack.
Gravelle, K., & Haskins, C. (1989). *Teenagers face to face with bereavement.* New York: Messner.
Grollman, E. (1993). *Straight talk about death for teenagers.* Boston: Beacon Press.
Hermes, P. (1982). *You shouldn't have to say goodbye.* New York: Scholastic.
Mahon, K. A. (1992). *Just one tear.* New York: Lethrop, Lee, and Shepard.
Rodowsky, C. (1996). *Remembering Mog.* New York: Farrar, Straus and Giroux.
Saint-Exupery, A. (1943). *The little prince.* New York: Harcourt Brace.

For Children

Brown, L. K., & Brown, M. B. (1996). *When dinosaurs die: A guide to understanding death*. Boston: Little, Brown.

Clifton, L. (1983). *Everett Anderson's goodbye*. New York: Henry Holt.

Fry, V. L. (1995). *Part of me died, too*. New York: Dutton Children's Books.

Mellonie, B., & Ingpen, R. (1983). *Lifetimes: The beautiful way to explain death to children*. Toronto: Bantam.

Powell, E. (1990). *Geranium morning*. Minneapolis, MN: Carolrhoda Books.

Rofes, E. E. (1985). *The kids' book about death and dying: By and for kids*. New York: Little, Brown.

Viorst, J. (1971). *The tenth good thing about Barney*. New York: Aladdin.

For Caregivers

Doka, E. (Ed.). (1995). *Children mourning, mourning children*. Washington, DC: Hospice Foundation of America.

Fitzgerald, H. (1992). *The grieving child: A parent's guide*. New York: Simon and Schuster.

Kroen, W. C. (1996). *Helping children cope with the loss of a loved one: A guide for grownups*. Minneapolis, MN: Free Spirit.

Kübler-Ross, E. (1983). *On children and death*. New York: Touchstone

LaTour, K. (1983). *For those who live: Helping children cope with the death of a brother or sister*. Omaha, NE: Centering Corporation.

McCue, K. (1994). *How to help children through a parent's serious illness*. New York: St. Martin's Press.

Schaefer, D., & Lyons, C. (1986). *How do we tell the children?* New York: Newmarket Press.

Wass, H., & Corr, C. (Eds.). (1982). *Helping children cope with death: Guidelines and resources*. New York: Hemisphere Publishing.

Wass, H., & Corr, C. (1984). *Childhood and death*. New York: Hemisphere Publishing.

Webb, N. (Ed.). (1993). *Helping bereaved children: A handbook for practitioners*. New York: Guilford Press.

Wolfelt, A. (1983). *Helping children cope with grief*. Bristol PA: Accelerated Development.

26

Grief, Death, Loss, and Life

Betty J. Kramer

"Only the person who is incapable of loving another is entirely free of the possibility of grief."—Sister Monica Ann Lucas

COURSE OVERVIEW

Grief, death, loss, and bereavement are pervasive and fundamental aspects of the human experience. An understanding of the grief process and the ways in which social workers may facilitate this process is essential to effective social work practice in all settings and with all age groups. The purpose of this course is to introduce students to the nature and centrality of the experience of loss and subsequent grief in their personal lives, in the lives of their clients, and in their roles as professional helpers. Emphasis is placed on the variety and types of loss experienced throughout the life cycle and the ways in which social workers may address grief-related needs with individuals across the life span. Throughout the course, attention is given to cultural diversity and norms; the wide variation in the grief experience; the influence of the developmental phase of the life span; identification of interventions that are evidence based; and recognition of the capacities, resilience, and growth of individuals and families confronted with loss. Through explorations of the material, the course is designed to stimulate a deeper self-awareness, an ability to be more fully present, and increased skill in assisting others and ourselves through the grief process.

A key objective of the course is to allow students to determine their own learning needs. Thus, a variety of assignments from which students may choose an area of focus is provided. Students will be required to review the course assignments and turn in a learning contract indicating their choice of assignments and dates for completion by the second week of class.

COURSE OBJECTIVES

This course will teach students:

- To analyze the empirical support for the grief work hypothesis
- To examine the nature and universality of the experience of grief as a response to loss
- To explore one's own losses and develop an understanding of the importance of facing and dealing with one's own grief in order to be present for grieving clients
- To critically review current theories of grief, mourning, and bereavement and the cultural variations in the experience of grief
- To analyze the dynamics and tasks of the grieving/mourning process, the distinctions between healthy grieving and complicated mourning, and the various manifestations of grief (i.e., feelings, physical sensations, and behaviors)
- To examine the wide range and types of often-monumental losses experienced throughout the life cycle and by the varied populations served by social workers
- To become familiar with a variety of grief intervention modalities across the life span and to become aware of existing evidence about which methods are most effective for whom
- To explore writings on the near-death experience and develop an understanding of the special awareness, needs, and communications of the dying

REQUIRED TEXTS

Callanan, M., & Kelley, P. (1997). *Final gifts: Understanding the special awareness, needs, and communications of the dying*. New York: Bantam Books.
Hooyman, N. R., & Kramer, B. J. (2005). *Living through loss: Interventions across the lifespan*. New York: Columbia University Press.
Morse, M. (1990). *Closer to the light: Learning from the near-death experiences of children*. New York: Ivy Books.

COURSE REQUIREMENTS

Attendance and participation in class discussion and activities: Although a variety of learning methods will be incorporated, there will be an emphasis on critical discussion and class activities. Students are expected to assume responsibility for their own learning and show their progress by demonstrating mastery of the weekly readings and through active class participation.

Therefore, it is important that students complete the readings each week in preparation for class discussions.

In-class training workshop

Completion of a major paper (e.g., discussion of cultural variation in beliefs or practices; critical review of the theories of grief, mourning, or bereavement; analysis of evidence for or against the grief work hypothesis), a personal loss lifeline and reflection, an age-appropriate therapeutic tool, or a self-directed proposal

COURSE OUTLINE

*Required reading
**Recommended reading

Session 1 Introduction: Grief as a response to loss and its relevance to the profession
Types of losses
Understanding attitudes and societal response to loss/grief
The grief work hypothesis (empirical support for and against)

Reading:
*Hooyman & Kramer, introduction
**Murray, J. A. (2001). Loss as a universal concept: A review of the literature to identify common aspects of loss in diverse situations. *Journal of Loss and Trauma, 6,* 219–241.

Session 2 Theoretical perspectives on grief and self-awareness of personal losses
Definitions of key terms
Cultural differences
Classical paradigm of grief
Critique of the grief work hypothesis
The social worker's self-examination; personal reflections
The impact of professional grief

Reading:
*Hooyman, & Kramer, chapter 1
**Fox, R., & Cooper, M. (1998). The effects of suicide on the private practitioner: A professional and personal perspective. *Clinical Social Work Journal, 17*(1), 55–64.
**Leff, P., Chan, J., & Walizer, E. (1991). Self-understanding and reaching out to sick children and their families: An ongoing professional challenge. *Children's Health Care, 20*(4), 230–239.
**Lindstrom, T. C. (2002). "It ain't necessarily so" . . . Challenging

mainstream thinking about bereavement. *Family Community Health, 25*(1), 11–21.

Session 3 The grief process
Tasks and phases of grief
Integrative and dual-process models of grief
Assessment and measurement of grief
What is complicated mourning?
Cultural competence
Resiliency framework

Reading:
*Hooyman & Kramer, chapters 2 and 3
**DeSpelder, L. A. (1998). Developing cultural competency. In K. J. Doka & J. D. Davidson (Eds.), *Living with grief: Who we are, how we grieve* (pp. 97–106). Washington, DC: Hospice Foundation of America.
**Klass, D. (1999). Developing a cross-cultural model of grief: The state of the field. *Omega: Journal of Death and Dying, 39*(3), 153–178.
**Stroebe, M. S., & Schut, H. (2001). Models of coping with bereavement: A review. In M. S. Stroebe, R. O. Hansson, W. Stroebe, & H. Schut (Eds.), *Handbook of bereavement research: consequences, coping and care* (pp. 375–403). Washington, DC: American Psychological Association.
**Tomita, T., & Kitamura, T. (2002). Clinical and research measures of grief: A reconsideration. *Comprehensive Psychiatry, 43*(2), 95–102.

Session 4 Losses experience in childhood
Developmental considerations
Resiliency model
Children and traumatic grief
Death of a parent, sibling, or other family member
Loss and adoption
Loss and foster care

Reading:
*Hooyman & Kramer, chapter 4
**Jenkins, E. J., & Bell, C. C. (1997). Exposure and response to community violence among children and adolescents. In J. D. Osofsky (Ed.), *Children in a violent society* (pp. 9–31). New York: Guilford Press.
**Matthews, J. D. (1999). The grieving child in the school environment. In J. D. Davidson & K. J. Doka (Eds.), *Living with*

grief: At work, at school, at worship (pp. 95–113). Washington, DC: Hospice Foundation of America.

**Oltjenbruns, K. A. (2001). Developmental context of childhood: Grief and regrief phenomena. In M. S. Stroebe, R. O. Hansson, W. Stroebe, & H. Schut (Eds.), *Handbook of bereavement research* (pp. 169–197). Washington, DC: American Psychological Association.

**Young, B., & Papadatou, D. (1997). Childhood death and bereavement across cultures. In C. M. Parkes, P. Laugani, & B. Young (Eds.), *Death and bereavement across cultures* (pp. 191–205). New York: Routledge.

**Zambelli, G. C., & Clark, E. J. (1994). Parentally bereaved children: Problems in school adjustment and implications for the school social worker. *School Social Work Journal, 19,* 1–15.

Session 5 Interventions for grieving children

Issues related to grief interventions with children

General techniques and interventions

Communication issues with grieving children; guidelines for breaking bad news

The importance of rituals

Mastery through play (cultural considerations in play therapy)

Group-, family-, and school-based interventions

Interventions for children exposed to specific losses

Pet death

Responding to traumatic events (traumatic bereavement, parental homicide, community- and school-based interventions)

Children in foster care; abused children

Reading:

*Hooyman & Kramer, chapter 5

**Bluestone, J. (1999). School-based peer therapy to facilitate mourning in latency-age children following sudden parental death. In N. B. Webb (Ed.), *Play therapy with children in crisis: Individual, group, and family treatment* (pp. 225–251). New York: Guilford Press.

**Doka, K. J. (2000). Using ritual with children and adolescents. In K. J. Doka (Ed.), *Living with grief: Children, adolescents, and loss* (pp. 153–159). Washington, DC: Hospice Foundation of America.

**Edelstein, S. B., Burge, D., & Waterman, J. (2001). Helping foster parents cope with separation, loss, and grief. *Child Welfare, 80*(1), 5–25.

**Goldman, L. (1996). Techniques for complicated grief. In *Breaking the silence: A guide to help children with compli-*

cated grief: Suicide, homicide, AIDS, violence, and abuse (pp. 93–116). Washington, DC: Accelerated Learning.
**Oppawsky, J. (1991). Utilizing children's drawings in working with children following divorce. *Journal of Divorce and Remarriage, 15*(3/4), 125–141.
**Webb, N. B. (2000). Play therapy to help bereaved children. In K. J. Doka (Ed.), *Living with grief: Children, adolescents, and loss* (pp. 139–152). Washington, DC: Hospice Foundation of America.

Session 6 Losses experienced in adolescence
Developmental consideration
Nature of adolescent grief
Death of family members
Divorce/separation
Death of peers (violence, homicide, suicide)
Adolescents as bereaved parents (abortion, miscarriage, relinquishing child for adoption)
Teen pregnancy/abortion

Reading:
*Hooyman, & Kramer, chapter 6
**Balk, D. E. (2000). Adolescents, grief, and loss. In K. J. Doka (Ed.), *Living with grief: Children, adolescents, and loss* (pp. 35–49). Washington, DC: Hospice Foundation of America.
**Christ, G. H., Siegel, K., & Christ, A. E. (2002). Adolescent grief: "It never really hit me . . . until it actually happened." *Journal of the American Medical Association, 288,* 1269–1279.
**Hogan, N., & DeSantis, L. (1994). Things that help and hinder adolescent sibling bereavement. *Western Journal of Nursing Research, 16*(2), 132–153.
**Joralemon, B. (1986). Terminating an adolescent pregnancy: Choice and loss. In C. Corr & J. McNeil (Eds.), *Adolescence and death* (pp. 119–131). New York: Springer.
**O'Brien, J., Goodenow, C., & Espin, O. (1991). Adolescents' reactions to the death of a peer. *Adolescence, 26,* 431–440.
**Schachter, S. (1991). Adolescent experiences with the death of a peer. *Omega: Journal of Death and Dying, 24,* 1–11.

Session 7 Interventions for grieving adolescents
Issues realted to grief interventions with teens
General techniques and interventions for grieving teens
Death education and grief supports in schools
Group-based interventions

Expressing grief through music
Counseling male adolescents
Interventions for adolescents exposed to specific losses
Death in the family, teen pregnancy, suicide (prevention, intervention, and postvention)
Trauma, community, and gang violence

Reading:
*Hooyman & Kramer, chapter 7
**Cohen, J. A., Greenberg, T., Padlo, S., Shipley, C. Mannarino, A. P., Deblinger, E., & Stubenbort, K. (2001). *Cognitive behavioral therapy for traumatic bereavement in children treatment manual.* Pittsburgh: Center for Traumatic Stress in Children and Adolescents.
**Gough, M. (2000). Smashing pumpkins and blind melons: Using popular music to help grieving adolescents. In J. D. Morgan (Ed.), *Meeting the needs of our clients creatively: The impact of art and culture on caregiving* (pp. 151–165). Amityville, NY: Baywood.
**O'Donnell, L., Stueve, A., Wardlaw, D., & O'Donnell, C. (2003). Adolescent suicidality and adult support: The reach for health study of urban youth. *American Journal of Health Behavior, 27,* 633–644.
**O'Halloran, M. (2000). Adjustment to parental separation and divorce. In A. Carr (Ed.), *What works with children and adolescents? A critical review of psychological interventions with children adolescents and their families* (pp. 280–299). Florence, KY: Taylor and Francis/Routledge.
**Saltzman, W. R., Pynoos, R. S., Layne, C. M., Steinberg, A. M., & Aisenberg, E. (2001). Trauma- and grief-focused intervention for adolescents exposed to community violence: Results of a school-based screening and group treatment protocol. *Group Dynamics: Theory, Research, and Practice, 5*(4), 291–303.
**Wilby, J. (1995). Transcultural counselling: Bereavement counselling with adolescents. In S. C. Smith & M. Pennells (Eds.), *Interventions with bereaved children* (pp. 232–240). London: Jessica Kingsley.

Session 8 Losses experienced in young adulthood
Developmental considerations
Resiliency
Death of a child (miscarriage, stillbirth, sudden infant death)
Abortion or relinquishing a child to adoption
Birth of a child with disabilities

Death of a partner
HIV/AIDS
Physical and sexual abuse

Reading:
*Hooyman & Kramer, chapter 8
**Chew, J. (1998). Living through the legacy: Childhood sexual abuse—a working definition. In *Women survivors of childhood sexual abuse: Healing through group work* (pp. 3–15). New York: Haworth Press.
**Corless, I. B. (1997). Modulating mourning: The grief and mourning of those infected and affected by HIV/AIDS. In K. J. Doka & J. Davidson (Eds.), *Living with grief when illness is prolonged* (pp. 105–117). Washington, DC: Hospice Foundation of America.
**Ellis, J. (1989). Grieving for the loss of the perfect child: Parents of children with handicaps. *Child and adolescent social work, 6*(4), 259–270.
**Hebert, M. P. (1998). Perinatal bereavement in its cultural context. *Death Studies, 22,* 61–78.
**Luchterhand, C., & Murphy, N. (1998). What is unique for adults with mental retardation. In *Helping adults with mental retardation grieve a death loss* (pp. 15–26). Bristol, PN: Accelerated Development.
**Seigerman, A. (2001). A social worker's perspective on pregnancy loss. In M. R. Berman (Ed.), *Parenthood lost: Healing pain after miscarriage, stillbirth, and infant death* (pp. 89–93). Westport, CT: Bergin and Garvey.

Session 9 Interventions for grieving young adults
Issues related to grief interventions with young adults
General techniques and intervention
Social support and group based interventions (support, Web-based support, and therapeutic bereavement groups), family-based interventions, creating healing rituals
Interventions for young adults exposed to specific losses
Perinatal death and other losses (abortion, miscarriage, stillbirth and neonatal death, SIDS, adoption)
Developmental disabilities, sexual or physical abuse, HIV/AIDS
Young widows and widowers

Reading:
*Hooyman & Kramer, chapter 9
**Becvar, D. S. (2001). Creating funerals, ceremonies, and other healing rituals. In *In the presence of grief: Helping family*

members resolve death, dying, and bereavement issues (pp. 207–225). New York: Guilford Press.

**Gray, S. W., Zide, M. R., & Wilker, H. (2000). Using the solution focused brief therapy model with bereavement groups in rural communities: Resiliency at its best. *Hospice Journal, 15*(3), 13–30.

**Johnson, S. (1987). Interventions. In *After a child dies* (pp. 153–185). New York: Springer.

**Kulic, K. R. (2003). An account of group work with family members of 9/11. *Journal of Specialists in Group Work, 28*(3), 195–198.

**Pauw, M. (1991). The social worker's role with a fetal demise and stillbirth. *Health and Social Work, 16*(4), 291–297.

**Reilly-Smorawski, B., Armstrong, A. V., & Catlin, E. A. (2002). Bereavement support for couples following death of a baby: Program development and 14-year exit analysis. *Death Studies, 26,* 21–37

Session 10 Losses experienced in midlife
Developmental consideration
Resiliency
Death of an adolescent/adult child
Divorce
Caring for an adult child with chronic mental illness
Caring for older relatives
Death of a parent

Reading:
*Hooyman & Kramer, chapter 10

**Eakes, G. (1995). Chronic sorrow: The lived experience of parents of chronically mentally ill individuals. *Archives of Psychiatric Nursing, 9*(2), 77–84.

**MacGregor, P. (1994). Grief: The unrecognized parental response to mental illness in a child. *Social Work, 39*(2), 160–166.

**Scharlach, A. E., & Fredriksen, K. I. (1993). Reactions to the death of parent during midlife. *Omega: Journal of Death and Dying, 27,* 301–317.

**Staudacher, C. (1991). Understanding men's grief responses. In *Men and grief: A guide for men surviving the death of a loved one: A resource for caregivers and mental health professionals* (pp. 11–41). Oakland, CA: New Harbinger Publications.

Session 11 Intervention for grieving midlife adults
Developmental considerations
Assessment, telling the story of a loss

General techniques and interventions
Grief counseling and therapy
Counseling techniques and cultural considerations
Interventions for midlife adults exposed to specific losses
Parents of children with life-threatening illness
Parents of a child who dies suddenly
Death of a parent
Divorce
Interventions for family caregivers

Reading:
*Hooyman & Kramer, chapter 11
**Canine, S. L. (1996). Counseling techniques for helping the bereaved. In *The psychosocial aspects of death and dying* (pp. 253–264). Stamford, CT: Appleton and Lange.
**Deranieri, J. T., Clements, P. T., & Henry, G. C. (2002). Assessment and intervention after sudden traumatic death. *Journal of Psychosocial Nursing, 40*(4), 30–37.
**Jordan, J. R., & Neimeyer, R. A. (2003). Does grief counseling work? *Death Studies, 27,* 765–786.
**Kissane, D. W., Bloch, S. McKenzie, M., McDowall, A. C., & Nitzan, R. (1998). Family grief therapy: A preliminary account of a new model to promote health family functioning during palliative care and bereavement. *Psycho-oncology, 7,* 14–25.
**Schwartz-Borden, G. (1992). Metaphor: Visual aid in grief work. *Omega: Journal of Death and Dying, 25*(3), 239–248.
**Sedney, M. A., Baker, J. E., & Gross, E. (1994). "The story" of a death: Therapeutic considerations with bereaved families. *Journal of Marital and Family Therapy, 20*(3), 287–296.

Session 12 Losses experienced in later life
Developmental considerations and nature of loss in later life
Resiliency
Death of a partner
Death of a friend
Death of a sibling
Caregiving in old age (caregivers of grandchildren, caring for adults with developmental disabilities)
Elder abuse and neglect
Chronic illness and pain

Reading:
*Hooyman & Kramer, chapter 12
**Arbore, P. (2002). Suicide in older people. In K. J. Doka (Ed.), *Living with grief: Loss in later life* (pp. 253–271). Washington, DC: Hospice Foundation of America.

**Blank, J. W. (1998). A summing up: Special problems of parents whose adult children died. In *The death of an adult child: A book for and about bereaved parents*. Amityville, NY: Baywood.

**Keay, T. J. (2002). Issues of loss and grief in long-term care facilities. In K. J. Doka (Ed.), *Living with grief: Loss in later life* (pp. 119–129). Washington, DC: Hospice Foundation of America.

**Loos, C., & Bowd, A. (1997). Caregivers of persons with Alzheimer's disease: Some neglected implications of the experience of personal loss and grief. *Death Studies, 21,* 501–514.

**Moss, M., Moss, S., & Hansson, R. (2001). Bereavement and old age. In M. S. Stroebe, R. O. Hansson, W. Stroebe, & H. Schut (Eds.), *Handbook of bereavement research: Consequences, coping, and care* (pp. 241–260). Washington, DC: American Psychological Association.

Session 13 Interventions for grieving older adults

Issues related to grief interventions with older adults
Communication and responding to grief of elders
Grief resurgence in later life
General techniques and interventions
Reminiscence and life review
Counseling and psychotherapy
Group work
Grief in older men
Spiritually attentive interventions
Interventions for elders exposed to specific losses
Spousal bereavement
Suicide
Dementia
Family caregiving
Life transitions
Grief and approaching death

Reading:

*Hooyman & Kramer, chapter 13

**Liken, M., & Collins, C. (1993). Grieving: Facilitating the process for dementia caregivers. *Journal of Psychosocial Nursing, 31*(1), 21–26.

**Molinari, V. (1999). Using reminiscence and life review as natural therapeutic strategies in group therapy. In M. Duffy (Ed.), *Handbook of counseling and psychotherapy with older adults* (pp. 154–165). New York: John Wiley and Sons.

**Nadeau, J. W. (2002). Counseling later-life families. In K. Doka (Ed.), *Living with grief: Loss in later life* (pp. 313–327). Washington, DC: Hospice Foundation of America.

**Zisook, S., & Shuchter, S. R. (2001). Treatment of the depressions of bereavement. *American Behavioral Scientist, 44*(5), 782–797.

Session 14 Hope, hospice, and healing
The work of hospice in addressing grief
Communications of the dying
Near-death awareness
Near-death experience
Growth through loss

Reading:
*Callanan & Kelley
*Morse
**Miller, S. C., Mor, V., Gage, B., & Coppola, K. (2000). Hospice and its role in improving end-of-life care. In M. P. Lawton (Ed.), *Annual Review of Gerontology and Geriatrics, 20* (pp. 193–223). New York: Springer.

Session 15 Professional self-care
Summary, integration, and evaluation
Burnout and causes of stress in practice
Class evaluation

Reading:
*Hooyman & Kramer, chapter 14
**DiGiulio, J. F. (1995). A more humane workplace: Responding to child welfare workers' personal losses. *Child Welfare, 74*(4), 877–888.

**Foster, Z., & Davidson, K. (1995). Satisfactions and stresses for the social worker. In I. B. Corless, B. B. Germino, & M. A. Pittman (Eds.), *Dying, death, and bereavement: A challenge for living* (pp. 285–300). Boston: Jones and Bartlett.

**McLeod, B. W. (2001). Self-care: The path to wholeness. In K. J. Doka (Ed.), *Caregiving and loss: Family needs, professional responses* (pp. 195–207). Washington, DC: Hospice Foundation of America.

**Wolfelt, A. D. (2001). How to care for yourself while you care for bereaved families. In O. D. Weeks & C. Johnson (Eds.), *When all the friends have gone: A guide for aftercare providers* (pp. 229–246). Amityville, NY: Baywood.

Learning Contract

I, ______________________________, agree to complete the following assignments by the dates indicated below. (NOTE: Consider when related course material will be covered in class so that you do not agree to turn in an assignment before we have covered the material.) Please make one copy for yourself and turn this top sheet in by the second week of class.

	Date To Be Completed
A. Required: (35 points)	
In-class training workshop	____________
The topic is: ____________________	
B. Choose One: (50 points)	____________
1. Major paper (e.g., discussion of cultural variation in beliefs, practices; critical review of the theories of grief, mourning, or bereavement; analysis of evidence for or against the grief work hypothesis)	____________
2. Personal loss lifeline and reflection	____________
3. Age-appropriate therapeutic tool	____________
4. Self-directed proposal	____________

____________________________________ ____________

Student Signature Date

IN-CLASS TRAINING WORKSHOP

This assignment allows you to work with other students to investigate one of the following: (1) a type of loss experienced by a particular client population (e.g., AIDS, chronic illness, abuse, separation, death, miscarriage); (2) a type of intervention, skill, or method that may be used to assist grieving clients (e.g., metaphor, play, drawing, school-based strategies, counseling, rituals, support groups); or (3) a related topic that you believe social workers should be well informed about (e.g., ethical or legal issues). Your team should thoroughly investigate the research and practice literature related to your chosen topic and then prepare a presentation that will inform other students about what you have learned.

The presentation should help students to understand the following:

- What do we know and not know about the topic (according to researchers and practitioners)? For example, you might consider the gaps in knowledge or the limitations of prior research.
- What primary theoretical frameworks inform what we know about the topic and how adequate are they?
- What are the implications for practice?

You should also attempt to develop exercises that will either sensitize students to the issues you are exploring (if it is a loss issue or special topic) or allow them to practice the skill in class. You are encouraged to be creative (e.g., write a play, sing a song, dramatize an event), to use teaching strategies that will enhance learning and make your topic interesting (e.g., handouts, films), and to think critically about the material you are examining. You may want to talk with practitioners in the community who know something about the topic to learn from their experiences. On the day of your presentation, you must provide a typed APA-style reference list for all in attendance. You need to provide full citations for all resources you used in your review of the literature and presentation planning so that students who wish to explore the topic further will know where to begin. Your presentation should be no longer than forty-five minutes.

MAJOR CRITICAL REVIEW PAPER

The purpose of this assignment is for you to critically review the current literature regarding a topic that is central to the objectives of this course. For example, you may want to compare and contrast cultural variations in beliefs or practices related to grief. Or you could investigate evidence for and against the grief work hypothesis. Or you could critically review the current theories of grief, mourning, or bereavement and discuss your theoretical preference and the rationale for your choice.

The task:

1. Select a topic central to the objectives of the course.
2. Write a thorough critical review of the literature relevant to your chosen topic. You should discuss what we know and do not know about the topic, providing evidence for and against your conclusions.
3. Conclude your paper with a discussion of the: (1) gaps in the literature, (2) limitations of prior research on the topic, (3) suggestions for future research, and (4) implications for social work practice.
4. Submit a paper of no more than fifteen pages. This should be written in APA style.

PERSONAL LOSS LIFELINE AND REFLECTION

The purpose of this assignment is to heighten your awareness of your personal losses and grieving style, to provide you with the opportunity to personally relate to the course readings, and to help you identify the ways in which these personal experiences may affect your practice.

The task:

1. Construct a loss lifeline. On poster board or paper, construct a personal loss lifeline that identifies calendar years (beginning at birth) for all significant losses that you can recall. This should include both death-related and nondeath-related losses. You should identify your date of birth and also your age at the time of each loss on your loss lifeline.
2. Reflect on the loss lifeline. Once you have identified each loss, take some time to explore each loss by thinking about what was happening at the time and how you responded to each loss. You might consider the following questions: What do you remember about the loss experience? What did you feel, and how did that change over time? How did you cope? How did you grieve? How did others in your environment respond to your grief, and how did that affect your experience? To what extent are you still experiencing grief, and where are you at in the process?
3. Make connections to course readings and content. Reflect upon the ways in which your experience with loss and your grief response relate to the course reading in terms of your age and development, the way that you coped with your loss, and how you grieved over time (i.e., relate it to theories of grief and theories of coping with grief). Determine your grieving style or any patterns you notice in how you respond to loss.
4. Use the following section headings in a fifteen-page report to address the following:

   Brief summary of losses: Briefly (1–3 pages) summarize your losses, noting the types and scope of losses you have experienced.

   Relevance and connection to course readings and content: The major portion of your paper (10–12 pages) should describe ways that you made connections to the course reading and content (cite relevant readings and content that relate to your experience, your age, level of development, coping response, how you grieved and theories of grief and your ability to cope with grief) and identifify which theoretical framework most closely resembles your experience, providing evidence for and against your conclusions. How did the readings illuminate your understanding of your loss/grief experiences?

   Professional implications: Reflect on the extent to which your own losses may affect how you relate to grieving clients and the extent to which they may influence your ability to be present and unbiased (Are there particular client situations that may be more challenging for you to work with given your history of loss? Have you identified any unresolved grief that may need to be addressed before you work with clients who are grieving?) This should be one to two pages.

DEVELOPING AN AGE-APPROPRIATE THERAPEUTIC TOOL

Over the course of the semester you will have the opportunity to learn about many different types of losses that occur across the life span, and you will be exposed to interventions that are developmentally appropriate and commonly employed. The purpose of this assignment is for you to develop a therapeutic tool or intervention that may be used with a particular client group you are interested in working with and that may build upon or complement other interventions.

The task:

1. Select a particular age group, client population, or type of loss.
2. Carefully review the literature on the special needs and developmental issues of the client group and the therapeutic interventions that are most appropriate for use with the specified client group. Consider what has been found to work or not work with the population. Note: In reviewing the literature, you must review empirical and knowledge-based journal articles. It is not acceptable to review the topic in a general way (e.g., using the Internet to get suggestions for responding to a particular type of loss).
3. Taking special needs and developmental issues into consideration, create and design a unique age- and client-appropriate therapeutic tool or intervention. For example, you may develop a community presentation, an educational group, an age- or loss-specific ritual, or an activity book or manual.
5. Summarize the process that you went through to develop the tool. Include a brief review of the literature on the special needs and developmental issues that you built your project upon. Provide your reasons for developing the tool or intervention. Explain how, when, where, and why it might be used most effectively.
6. Submit a paper of no more than fifteen pages, along with a reference list and the therapeutic tool you have developed.

SELF-DIRECTED PROPOSAL (DESIGN YOUR OWN ASSIGNMENT)

Social work courses are typically composed of individuals with a wide variety of interests and skill levels. Taking this into consideration, this project offers you the opportunity to design your own major assignment for this course. For example, some of you may have a particular interest in developing group work skills by facilitating an informational, supportive, or educational group related to grief. Others may have an interest in studying some type of intervention method to be used with clients. Yet others may be interested in conducting a research project related to the topic of grief.

You will need to draft a detailed proposal and present this to your instructor. Please keep in mind that the proposal should somehow be related to the course objectives. All proposals must be approved by your instructor.

27

Loss, Recovery, and Resilience

Froma Walsh

COURSE DESCRIPTION AND OBJECTIVES

This course will present a developmental systemic framework for understanding the individual and family impact and recovery processes that accompany the death of a loved one and other traumatic losses (e.g., separation/divorce, foster care and adoption, violence, community disaster, war-related trauma). Of all human experiences, death and loss pose the most painful challenges for adaptation. The course will first address end-of-life issues, including ethical decision-making dilemmas. It will then focus on bereavement and recovery processes and their application to other losses. We will examine how risk factors and unresolved loss can contribute to a range of dysfunctions (e.g., depression, relational difficulties, substance abuse, and children's behaviorial problems).

We will explore the loss of a parent, child, sibling, spouse, and other significant relationships at various family life-cycle stages, examining risk variables in (1) the nature and timing of losses; (2) family roles, relationship dynamics, and multigenerational legacies; and (3) diverse sociocultural and religious/spiritual influences. A research-informed family resilience framework will be applied to identify variables that foster resilience, healing, and growth. Practice guidelines will be offered for working collaboratively with individuals, couples, and families facing threatened loss, recent loss, and long-term complications. Lectures will be supplemented by film and case illustrations.

A multisystemic perspective will also inform discussion of ways (1) to advocate resources, policies, and practices that meet the needs of vulnerable and disenfranchised populations; (2) to work collaboratively for health-care and other larger systems to become more responsive to individual and family needs and concerns with death and loss; and (3) to seek opportunities to take activist positions to advance social change in organizations, communities, and society to lower the risk of traumatic death and loss (e.g., gun control) and to foster resilience for dealing with traumatic losses.

REQUIRED TEXTS

Walsh, F. (1998). *Strengthening family resilience.* New York: Guilford Press.
Walsh, F., & McGoldrick, M. (2004). *Living beyond loss: Death in the family* (2nd ed.). New York: W. W. Norton.
Worden, J. W. (2002). *Grief counseling and grief therapy: A handbook for the mental health practitioner* (3rd ed.). New York: Springer.

RECOMMENDED TEXTS

Rando, T. (Ed.). (1991). *Treatment of complicated mourning.* Champaign, IL: Research Press.
Rando, T. (Ed.). (1986). *Parental loss of a child.* Champaign, IL: Research Press.
Rolland, J. R. (1994). *Families, illness, and disability: An integrative treatment model.* New York: Basic Books.
Walsh, F. (Ed.). (1999). *Spiritual resources in family therapy.* New York: Guilford Press.
Walsh, F. (Ed.). (2003). *Normal family processes: Growing diversity and complexity* (3rd ed.). New York: Guilford Press.
Worden, J. W. (1996). *Children and grief.* New York: Guilford Press.

COURSE OUTLINE

* Required reading

Session 1 — Death and loss: An overview
Sociohistorical and multicultural perspectives on death and bereavement
Developmental, multisystemic orientation
Continuous bonds, varied pathways versus traditional views of bereavement
Individual and family adaptational challenges: Vulnerability, risk, and resilience

Reading:
*Walsh & McGoldrick, chapters 1 and 7
*Walsh (1998), chapter 1
Worden (2002), chapters 1 and 2

Session 2 — Loss and the family life cycle
Loss of older parent, life partner, other significant relationship
Film: *The Long Good-bye*
Untimely losses: Loss of a parent in childhood; loss of a child or sibling

Reading:
*Walsh & McGoldrick, chapters 2, 3, and 11

*Walsh & McGoldrick, section 3 (select 4):
Walsh, "Personal Reflections on loss"
McGoldrick, "Loss and Transformation"
Menos, "Tell Me She's Not Dead: Living beyond the Loss of Our Child"
Klages, "Different in the World: Hidden Dimensions of Sibling Loss"
Llerena-Quinn, "Naming the Tears: Loss in Cross-Cultural Context"
Garcia Preto, "Their Good Spirits Came to Take Them"
DeFrain, J. (1991). Learning about grief from normal families: SIDS, stillbirth, and miscarriage. *Journal of Marital and Family Therapy, 17,* 215–232.
Rando (1986)
Worden (1996)

Session 3 Facing death and loss: Application of resilience framework
Intervention priorities and guidelines
Being fully present; facilitating important conversations
Adaptational challenges and pathways in recovery from loss
Culture, class, and gender issues
Spiritual beliefs and rituals
Family dynamics; multigenerational legacies
Impact of unresolved past loss
Film: *Legacy of Loss*

Reading:
*Walsh & McGoldrick, chapters 4, 9, 16
*Walsh (1998), chapters 3 and 7
*Worden (2002), chapter 3
Walsh & McGoldrick, chapter 6

Session 4 Complicated loss: Variables in risk and resilience
Suicide, homicide, family and community violence
Belief systems: Blame, shame, guilt, and stigma/secrecy
Spiritual beliefs and practices: Meaningful rituals, faith communities; social action
Issues of reconciliation and forgiveness; justice in wrongful deaths
Facilitating healing, reconciliation, forgiveness
Film: *A Justice that Heals*

Reading:
*Walsh & McGoldrick, chapters 13 and 15
*Worden (2002), chapters 4 and 5

*Walsh (1998), chapter 10
Walsh & McGoldrick, section 3:
*Treadway, "People Die; Relationships Don't: Surviving My Mother's Suicide"
Jackson, "Surviving My Sister's Suicide: A Journey through Grief"
Walsh & McGoldrick, chapters 5 and 8
Rando (1991)

Session 5 Traumatic loss and resilience in major disaster, war, genocide, terrorism
Individual, family, and community recovery
Immediate and long-term impact
Facilitating coping and adaptation
Resilience-oriented programs for family and community recovery
Multifamily groups for Bosnian and Kosovar refugees
Kosovar professional training collaborative: Recovery in war-torn region
Post-9/11 Lower Manhattan Recovery Project; LINC model
Film: *Angels Too Soon*

Reading:
Handouts: Disaster preparedness; coping guidelines for children and families
*Walsh & McGoldrick, chapter 14
*Walsh & McGoldrick, section 3:
Rolland, "Family Legacies of the Holocaust"
Sluzki, "Hin und Zurück: Back to Where We Came From"
*Walsh, F. (2002). Bouncing forward: Resilience in the aftermath of September 11. *Family process, 40*(1), 34–36.
Nader, K. (1997). Childhood traumatic loss: The interaction of trauma and grief. In C. R. Figley, B. E. McBride, & N. Mazza (Eds.), *Death and trauma: The traumatology of grieving* (pp. 17–41). Washington, DC: Taylor and Francis.
Nader, K. (1997). Treating traumatic grief in systems. In C. R. Figley, B. E. McBride, & N. Mazza (Eds.), *Death and trauma: The traumatology of grieving* (pp. 159–192). Washington, DC: Taylor and Francis.

Session 6 Separation, divorce, foster care, adoption, migration
Linking and transforming vital connections
Loss and abandonment issues; facilitating reconnection, healing
Film: *First Person Plural*
Discussion of students' own family migration experiences: Losses, adaptational challenges, resilience

Reading:
*Minuchin, P., Colapinto, J., & Minuchin, S. (1998). Foster care: An ecological model. In *Working with families of the poor* (pp. 91–128). New York: Guilford Press.
*Walsh (2003), chapters 4, 8, and 11
*Walsh, F., Jacob, L., & Simon, V. (1995). Facilitating healthy divorce processes: Therapy and mediation approaches. In N. Jacobson & A. Gurman (Eds.), *Clinical handbook of couple therapy* (pp. 340–365). New York: Guilford Press.

Session 7 Terminal illness: Anticipatory loss, end-of life issues
Guest lecturer
Psychosocial challenges for patients, couples, and families
Impact of past illness and loss: Beliefs and catastrophic fears
Decision making: Ethical dilemmas, euthanasia, assisted suicide
Film cases and discussion

Reading:
*Walsh & McGoldrick, chapter 10
*Walsh & McGoldrick, section 3:
Carter, "My Father's Terminal Illness: Seizing the Moment for Change"
Reibstein, "My Family Inheritance of Breast Cancer"
*Walsh (1999), chapter 3
Rolland (1994)

Session 8 Living and dying with HIV/AIDS
Guest lecturer
Clinical practice issues: Unacknowledged and stigmatized losses
Film: *Strong Spirit Program: HIV/AIDS Men's Group*

Reading:
*Walsh & McGoldrick, chapter 12

Session 9 Combat-related trauma, stigma, guilt; long-term complications
Treatment approaches and barriers
Addressing couple and family strains
Film
Guest speaker
Final paper due for graduating students

Session 10 Personal/professional interface issues
Professional strains, compassion fatigue, resilience in working with loss
Clinician's own family experiences with loss; facing mortality
Dealing with loss issues in termination of therapy, other endings

Legacies of traumatic loss: Healing and resilience
Film: *Spirit with a Broken Heart*

Reading:
*Walsh & McGoldrick, chapter 17
*Worden (2002), chapter 8
*Walsh (1999), chapter 14

ASSIGNMENTS

Journal (sessions 1–8): Write a weekly reflection (1–2 pages, typed) after each class to facilitate integration of readings and classroom material.

Final term paper option 1: Applying a systemic perspective, examine salient loss issues, complications, recovery, and resilience in one of the following films: *Death in America, Hotel Rwanda, One True Thing, The Joy Luck Club, The Color Purple, Steel Magnolias, Longtime Companion, I Never Sang for My Father, Terms of Endearment,* or *Ponette.* Work in teams of two to three people in order to benefit from multiple perspectives and enrich the learning process. Once you have viewed the film, discuss it together; and draw on course readings, lectures, and class discussion to address the following:

- Discuss key relationships and family/community processes, strengths, and vulnerabilities surrounding loss. Note resiliencies in dealing with the loss. Where experience was traumatic, suggest how the family, social network/community, or others (and, as appropriate, a social worker) were or might be helpful in fostering healing and resilience.
- Briefly note developmental life-cycle issues (age, stage at loss, concurrent challenges, long-term legacies), as fitting.
- Discuss influences of gender, class, culture, race/ethnicity, spirituality, and the larger social/systemic/political context.
- Reflect briefly on your own personal/professional reactions and interface issues.

Final term paper option 2: You may instead choose to write a paper individually on a topic of interest to you (e.g., death of a child, parent loss, suicide, AIDS) with the approval of the instructor. Applying a developmental systemic perspective and drawing on relevant course readings, lectures, and class discussion, discuss the salient issues involving loss, recovery, and resilience.

28

Loss and Grief

Katherine Walsh

COURSE DESCRIPTION

This course is offered as a distance learning course. It prepares the MSW student for social work practice with clients coping with loss and grief. The initial focus increases students' awareness of, and sensitivity to, issues related to death, dying, disability, and grief related to loss. Theories of attachment and loss are used as a framework for assessing grief reactions in clients in different developmental stages and from different cultural backgrounds. Therapeutic interventions are examined and applied through case discussions and experiential exercises. (EPAS advanced curriculum content 4.0, 4.1, 4.2, 4.3, 4.5)

OBJECTIVES

Weekly journal entries, required responses in the threaded discussion, and a final exam will be used to assess students' mastery of the learning objectives. Upon completion of this course students will be able to:

- Identify their own personal philosophy and issues regarding death and loss and how these may affect their work with individuals and families experiencing loss (EPAS objectives 3.1.3, M6)
- Identify and understand normal grief and factors that contribute to unresolved loss and complicated bereavement (EPAS objectives 3.1.4, 3.1.7)
- Describe the impact of different types of losses at different stages of the life cycle (EPAS objective 3.1.7)
- Demonstrate sensitivity to, and awareness of, social and cultural attitudes and practices related to death and loss and describe how these influence coping with grief (EPAS objectives 3.1.1, 3.1.3)
- Describe diverse therapeutic interventions, including individual grief therapy and bereavement counseling as well as support groups and the circumstances in which they may be used effectively (EPAS objective M6)

- Demonstrate increased comfort as well as knowledge about death, loss, and grief (EPAS objectives 3.1.1, 3.1.2)

METHODS OF INSTRUCTION

The methods of instruction include independent reading and viewing of films; weekly entries into the class and team-teacher discussions; and review of lecture notes, handouts, and Internet resources. In addition, students will complete weekly integrative journal assignments and a final exam.

Journal: Students will keep a written integrative journal every week throughout the course. Journal entries can be drawn upon for online team-teacher discussions and class discussions as well as the exam. The journal is the student's learning tool and will consist of reflections on the readings and audiovisual supplements and students' own practice with clients. For some journal entries there will be assigned exercises from the text. It is expected that students will complete a journal entry each week for their own learning.

Online team-teacher discussions: The courseware allows for both a class discussion and a team-teacher discussion. These operate as asynchronous bulletin boards for online discussion and are a very important learning tool for the class. (This means students can submit entries at any time during the week, and they will be posted for course participants to view when they log in.) The members of the class will each be assigned to one of three small team-teacher discussion groups of five students each. The team-teacher discussion questions for each module are listed in the syllabus; however, the instructor will post the discussion questions for each team each week in the team-teacher discussion. Each week, students will enter their responses to the assigned questions in the team-teacher discussion. The questions will require students to reflect on their learning and apply concepts they have studied to case examples in the readings, audiovisual supplements, and/or (disguised) examples from students' own practice. Students are also encouraged to respond to a teammate's response or the instructor's response. Each student can only read the responses of members of his or her own team. However, the instructor will be asking students for permission to post exemplary responses to the class discussion, which everyone can read. Responses will be evaluated by the instructor based on the content mastery they reflect.

REQUIRED TEXT

Walsh-Burke, K. (2006). *Grief and loss: Theories and skills for helping professionals*. Needham Heights, MA: Allyn and Bacon.

RECOMMENDED TEXTS

Berzhoff, J., & Silverman, P. (2004). *Living with dying: A handbook for end-of-life healthcare practitioners*. New York: Columbia University Press.

Callahan, B. N. (1999). *Grief counseling: A manual for social workers*. Denver, CO: Love Publishing.

Crosson-Tower, C. (2003). *From the eye of the storm: The experiences of a child welfare worker*. Needham, MA: Allyn and Bacon (chapters 4 and 5).

Fry, V. (1995). *Part of me died too: Stories of creative survival among bereaved children and teenagers*. New York: Dutton Children's Books.

Gunther, J. (1998). *Death be not proud*. New York: HarperPerennial.

Krementz, J. (1988). *How it feels when a parent dies*. New York: Knopf.

Lerner, G. (1978). *A death of one's own*. New York: Harper and Row.

Mannino, J. D. (1997). *Grieving days, healing days*. Needham Heights, MA: Allyn and Bacon.

McGoldrick, M. (1991). *Living beyond loss*. London: W. W. Norton.

Rando, T. A. (1984). *Grief, dying and death*. Champaign, IL: Research Press.

Worden, J. W. (2002). *Grief counseling and grief therapy: A handbook for the mental health practitioner* (3rd ed.). New York: Springer.

AUDIOVISUAL SUPPLEMENTS

The distance learning format of this course enables students to view films, listen to audiotapes, and utilize interactive Internet-based resources at your home or office. A variety of films and tapes are suggested; these can be rented or borrowed from your local rental supplier or public library, or purchased online. Items marked with an asterisk (*) are recommended for the module. More than one option is listed for each week. Students may choose from the lists provided for each module and use your selection for online discussions and/or journal assignments.

A cautionary note regarding course material: The readings, exercises, and supplementary materials have been chosen for their themes of loss, which are relevant to the topic of the course. However, some of the material may elicit unanticipated emotional reactions. There may also be material in some of the supplementary audiovisual recommendations that some viewers may find objectionable. This is one of the reasons students are offered a choice of films. Students should exercise discretion and self-care in making choices and completing course assignments.

COURSE OUTLINE

Session 1 Review of symbolic loss and loss associated with death and dying
Self-evaluation

Reading:
Walsh-Burke, preface and chapter 1

Film: *Lorenzo's Oil, Spitfire Grill, Angela's Ashes, Kramer vs. Kramer, Seabiscuit, Antwone Fisher,* and *Stepmom* are films that address symbolic loss. Choose one and think about how the characters manifest grief in reaction to symbolic losses

Journal: Visit http://www.pbs.org/wnet/onourownterms/tools/index.html and complete both assessment tools: "Self-Assessment of Your Beliefs about Death" (under patient tools) and "Test Your Knowledge." Discuss your reactions to what you have learned from completing these tools.

Team-teacher discussion: Complete the exercise for chapter 1, p. 11. Share your responses to the exercise with your teammates by clicking on the team-teacher discussion posting for week 1.

Session 2 Exploring personal reactions to death, other losses, and grief
How do we feel about death and loss and working with clients affected by loss?

Reading: Walsh-Burke, chapter 2

Film: Choose any film related to loss that you have watched previously in your life that caused you to react emotionally. Be aware as you watch it this time how and why this film connects you to feelings related to loss. Try to assess what your reactions might be to working with clients who present these kinds of loss issues in the future.

Journal: In addition to writing briefly about your reactions to the assigned readings, complete the exercise at the end of chapter 2 (p. 26).

Team-teacher discussion: Enter your responses to the last question of the assigned exercise for chapter 2 into your team-teacher discussion. (How do you think your own feelings and reactions to loss may affect your work with others who are experiencing loss or trauma?)

Session 3 Loss and grief across the life span

Reading:
Walsh-Burke, chapter 3
Appendix A: Common losses across the life span
Appendix C: Annotated bibliography

Film: *Ponette, My Girl, My Life as a House, Antwone Fisher, Soul Food, Philadelphia, Dad,* and *Tuesdays with Morrie* all address grief in people at different life stages. Choose one, and note how what you have read in the assigned readings or at the Web sites you have visited is illustrated or contradicted in the film you chose.

Journal: In addition to briefly writing your reactions to the assigned readings, complete the exercise at the end of chapter 3 (pp. 41–42). Choose one of the stages of development discussed in the chapter (e.g., early childhood, adolescence, middle adulthood) to research online; visit Internet sites and read the material provided related to different developmental stages (e.g., children's grief, teen grief). Create your own archive of Web sites that you have found useful.

Team-teacher discussion: Choose three of the Internet sites you identified in completing the exercise for chapter 3 and share them with your teammates. Describe the content and format that you found helpful on these sites. Provide recommendations for your teammates about when and why they, or their clients, might use these sites. (At the completion of this week's team-teacher discussion, you will have a very useful collection of recommended Web sites.) These sites, along with the descriptions you provide for them, will be compiled and posted in the class discussion module so everyone will have a full list at the conclusion of the module.

Session 4 Normal and complicated grief

Reading:

Walsh-Burke, chapter 4

National Cancer Institute. (n.d.). *Loss, grief, and bereavment: Overview*. Available at http://www.cancer.gov/cancerinfo/pdq/supportivecare/bereavement/HealthProfessional

National Cancer Institute. (n.d.). *Loss, grief, and bereavment: Phases of bereavement*. Available at http://www.cancer.gov/cancertopics/pdq/supportivecare/bereavement/Health Professional/page5

National Cancer Institute. (n.d.). *Loss, grief, and bereavment: Complicated grief*. Available at http://www.cancer.gov/cancer topics/pdq/supportivecare/bereavement/HealthProfessional/page7

Journal: Complete parts 1 and 2 of the exercise at the end of chapter 4 (pp. 59–60). Think of someone you know who has experienced the death of a significant other. Using the normal emotions of grief as a checklist, note whether the person showed the signs of sadness, anger, or guilt that are part of normal grief. Describe your observations and note why you think he or she has evidenced normal or complicated grief.

Film: Choose a movie to watch (**Corinna, Corinna; Fearless; *Ponette; Smoke Signals; Life as a House;* or *Garden State*). As you view the movie, note the signs of complicated grief you observe.

Team-teacher discussion: Review part 3 of the exercise on p. 60. Enter your observations about a character in the film you selected (or describe a client on your own caseload), and describe why the grief the individual is evidencing is complicated. Describe what tasks of grieving were not completed that may have contributed to the complicated grief.

Session 5 Overview of interventions for normal and complicated grief

Reading:

Walsh-Burke, chapter 4

Walsh-Burke, K. (2000). Matching bereavement services to level of need. *Hospice Journal, 15*(1), 77–86.

General aspects of grief therapy

Journal: Review your journal entry for the overview of interventions for normal and complicated grief. Discuss what type of intervention(s) you might recommend to the individual you identified, why you would recommend these (for example, take into consideration the person's age, developmental stage, gender, and type of loss experience), and how you would present your recommendation to the person if you were a social worker working with him or her.

Team-teacher discussion: Discuss with your teammates what you have learned thus far about symbolic and actual loss and how you are applying grief theory differently now than you have in the past. Using your journal entry, discuss which of the interventions that you would recommend to the client or film case example are actually available to grieving clients in the agency or community in which you practice (e.g., Are there groups available to children, teens, adults? Are there experienced grief therapists to whom you could refer the individual or family? What online groups or referral sources have you identified, and could your clients access these?).

Session 6 Cultural and spiritual influences and grief

Reading: Walsh-Burke, chapter 5

Film: *Soul Food, *My Girl, Ordinary People, Smoke Signals, Steel Magnolias, Garden State,* or *To Live!*

Journal: In addition to writing your reactions to the assigned readings, complete the exercise for chapter 5 on p. 73.

Team-teacher discussion: Think about funerals, memorial services, or rituals of remembrance you have observed or in which you have participated that have seemed particularly helpful for those experiencing a loss. What aspects of these were similar to the practices of your own ethnic or religious group? What aspects were different? How do you feel about attending the funeral or memorial services of clients you work with?

Session 7 Individuals and families facing death

Reading:

Taylor-Brown, S., et al., Blacker, S., Walsh-Burke, K., Christ, G., & Altilio, T. (2001). *Social work and end of life care.* Best Practices Series. Philadelphia: Society for Social Work Leadership in Health Care.

National Cancer Institute. (n.d.). *Loss, grief, and bereavement: Model of life-threatening illness.* Available at http://www.cancer.gov/cancertopics/pdq/supportivecare/bereavement/HealthProfessional/page2

National Cancer Institute. (n.d.). *Loss, grief, and bereavement: The dying trajectory.* Available at http://www.cancer.gov/cancertopics/pdq/supportivecare/bereavement/HealthProfessional/page3

National Cancer Institute. (n.d.). *Loss, grief, and bereavement: Anticipatory grief.* Available at http://www.cancer.gov/cancertopics/pdq/supportivecare/bereavement/HealthProfessional/page4

Americans for Better Care for the Dying has published excerpts from this J. Lynne J. Harrold's *Handbook for mortals.* Go to http://www.abcd-caring.org/educate/index.html, and click on the book and then on "Read online excerpts." Then click on chapter 10, "Planning Ahead (Advance Care Planning)."

Film: *My Life* or *Tuesdays with Morrie*

Journal: After completing the readings, review the advance directives laws in your state (you can request forms for your state at http://www.caringinfo.org/i4a/forms/form.cfm?id=16andpageid=3462). Attach the forms or cut and paste them and write your own description of your state's laws in your journal entry. Discuss whether or not you have completed your own advance directives and why (or why not). Also discuss whether you have worked with clients around the issue of advance directives and what client situations you are involved in that might (now or in the future) require discussion of this by you, the social worker, or another helping professional.

Team-teacher discussion: When this course was offered previously, many students were interested in discussing the Terry Schiavo case (the comatose woman in Florida whose husband and parents were seeking different decisions from the court regarding the continuation of life support) and recommended that discussion of advance directives and the social work role in advance directives be included in this course. What role do you think you, as a social worker, have in discussing advance directives and end-of-life decision making with your clients? How do your own spiritual, cultural, and personal beliefs and coping strategies influence your thinking and actions in this area of practice? Do you agree with the previous students' recommendation that this content be included in this course?

Session 8 Misconceptions about grief
Helpful strategies for coping with grief
Utilizing resources

Reading:
Walsh-Burke, chapter 6
Appendix C: Helpful strategies for coping with grief
Appendix D: Strategies for professionals helping children and families with traumatic losses
Appendix F: Expressive techniques
Taplow, A. B. (1997). *Bereavement support group: Plans, handouts & notes*. Available at http://www.geocities.com/Tokyo/Towers/6662/berintro.htm

Recommended reading:
Worden, chapters 3 and 5

Film: **Ordinary People*, **Antwone Fisher*, *Legacy of Loss*, or *Teens Healing at Camp Braveheart*

Journal: Complete the exercise for chapter 6 on empathic listening. (You may ask a friend, classmate, or family member to complete the exercise with you.) In your journal, discuss your reactions to the exercise. Enter your answers to question 3 (How did it feel to be either the speaker or listener?) and question 5 (Discuss what the conversation was like in your new role).

Team-teacher discussion: After viewing *Ordinary People*, *Antwone Fisher*, *Teens Healing at Camp Braveheart*, or *Legacy of Loss,* write an assessment of the interventions you observed the counselor or group facilitator using in the film you selected, and discuss his or her effectiveness in addressing the needs of the grieving client(s). Discuss what concerns you have about the therapeutic approaches used or not used by the therapist/counselor. Discuss therapeutic interventions or approaches you might incorporate into your work with clients or family members in similar situations.

Session 9 Taking a leadership role
Establishing a bereavement protocol in your practice setting

Reading:
Walsh-Burke, chapter 7
Appendix E: Remembrance celebrations: Planning your own memorial service
Read the materials recommended in Internet Resources at http://www.nea.org/crisis and http://www.hospicefoundation.org

Film: *Stepmom, *Lorenzo's Oil, Soul Food, Longtime Companion, Saving Private Ryan,* or *Simon Birch*

Journal: Complete the exercise at the end of chapter 7, "Mapping a Bereavement Protocol for Your Organization."

Team-teacher discussion: Drawing on the assigned readings and the film you watched, which situations do you think would be the most challenging for you if you encountered them in your community or practice setting? Discuss why it might be challenging for you or others. Discuss what issues it might be useful for you to work on so that you will be able to be helpful in those situations in a practice setting.

Session 10 Professional support systems
Self-care strategies
Continuing education

Reading:
Walsh-Burke, chapter 8
Appendix G: Caregivers retreat agenda

Journal: Write your reflections on this week's readings and your study of grief and loss as a whole in this course. Complete the exercise for this chapter on p. 102.

Team-teacher discussion: Share your answer to the last question in the exercise: What plans do you have to sustain yourself in your work with grieving clients in the future? What strategies and methods do you plan to use personally to prevent burnout and compassion fatigue, and to maintain a balance in your professional and personal life?

Session 11 Reflections on what you have learned from this course

Journal: Reflect on what you learned from this course that you have already begun applying in your social work practice and/or your own personal life in relation to symbolic losses, actual losses, or both. How will what you have learned influence your work as a social worker or your approach as a family member, co-worker, or friend?

Team-teacher discussion: Reflect on a client you wrote about earlier in the course, a case you wrote about in a previous class, a grief situation in a film that you viewed, or a personal situation related to grief that you might encounter in the future. Describe what the difference is between how you would have approached this situation prior to taking this course and the approach that you would use now that you have completed the course and are looking through the lens of loss and grief. Include any relevant literature, class exercises, or resources that have influenced your thinking.

BIBLIOGRAPHY

Bullis, R. K. (1996). *Spirituality in social work practice.* Washington, DC: Taylor and Francis.

Cline, R. J. W., & Boyd, M. F. (1993). Communication as threat and therapy: Stigma, social support, and coping with HIV infection. In E. B. Ray (Eds.), *Case studies in health communication* (pp. 365–386). Hillsdale, NJ: Lawrence Erlbaum.

Corr, C., & Corr, D. (Eds.). (1983). *Hospice care: Principles and practice.* New York: Springer.

Corwin, M. D. (1995). Cultural issues in bereavement therapy: The social construction of mourning. *Psychotherapy in Practice, 1*(4), 23–41.

Cowley, A. S., & Derezotes, D. (1994). Transpersonal psychology and social work education. *Journal of Social Work Education, 30*(1), 32–41.

Dhooper, S. S. (1997). *Social work in health care in the 21st century.* Thousand Oaks, CA: Sage.

Doka, K. J. (1993). *Living with life-threatening illness: A guide for patients, their families, and caregivers.* San Francisco: Jossey-Bass.

Holland, J. C. (Ed.). (1998). *Psycho-oncology.* New York: Oxford University Press.

Kastenbaum, R. (2004). *Death, society and human experience.* Needham Heights, MA: Allyn and Bacon.

Last Acts. (2001). *Diversity and end of life care.* Retrieved August 2005 from http://lastacts.org/files/publications/Diversity1.15.02.pdf

Leming, M. R., & Dickinson, G. E. (2002). *Understanding dying, death, and bereavement* (5th ed.). New York: Harcourt College.

Lynne, J., & Harrold, J. (1999). *Handbook for mortals.* Washington, DC: Americans for Better Care for the Dying.

Padatou, D., & Papadatos, C. (Eds.). (1991). *Children and death*. New York: Hemisphere Publishing.

Stearns, N., Lauria, M., Hermann, J., & Fogelberg, P. (1993). *Oncology social work: A clinician's guide*. Atlanta, GA: American Cancer Society.

Stringham, J. G., Riley, J. H., & Ross, A. (1982). Silent birth: Mourning a stillborn baby. *Social Work*, 322–326.

Toolkit for Change. (2000–2006). *Competence assessments for professionals and organizations providing end of life care*. Retrieved from http://www.supportivecare coalition.org/ToolsExcellence/assessment_tools

Wells, P. J. (1993). Preparing for sudden death: Social work in the emergency room. *Social Work, 38*(3), 339–342.

Part Eight

MSW Specialty Course Syllabi

29

Introduction to Nursing Homes

Mercedes Bern-Klug

COURSE DESCRIPTION

With changes in reimbursement, demography, and illness trends, the role that nursing homes occupy in American society continues to evolve. In general, contemporary nursing homes provide services for three groups of people: those in need of subacute post-hospital care, those in need of care for chronic illnesses on a long-term basis, and those with end-of-life care needs. Therefore, the nursing home setting is one of rehabilitation, daily living, and care for people who are approaching death.

At the end of 2002, there were about 17,000 nursing homes in the United States, 16,471 of which were certified to accept Medicare and/or Medicaid reimbursements. Almost two-thirds of certified nursing homes are for-profit. The remaining third are not-for-profit or government sponsored, according to the Web site of the American Association of Homes and Services for the Aging.

This course presents an overview of the role of nursing homes within the context of the long-term care system. The course focuses on the concepts of quality of care and quality of life. The characteristics of people who live in nursing homes and the roles of key nursing home staff members, residents, and family members will be discussed. The course concludes by reviewing alternative nursing home models.

OBJECTIVES

The goal of this course is for students to

- Develop a basic understanding of the long-term care system in the United States, and the role of nursing homes within that system
- Understand the diversity of people who live in nursing homes and gain awareness of significant issues related to living and dying in the nursing home context
- Develop an appreciation for the key staff roles in nursing homes and the competing concerns faced by staff members as they do their work

- Recognize major developments in the attempt to assess and improve quality of care and quality of life in the nursing home setting
- Become familiar with classic research and policy documents regarding nursing homes in the United States
- Be prepared to critically evaluate and put into context developments in medical and social research related to nursing homes

At the end of the semester course, students will be able to:

- Describe institutional and noninstitutional long-term care settings
- Analyze the role that nursing homes play in U.S. society
- Contrast the physical, cognitive, and social needs of people who use long-term care and nursing home services
- Synthesize past and current attempts to assess and enhance the quality of care and quality of life provided in the nursing home setting
- Describe the role of at least three nursing home staff members
- Compare and contrast alternate models for long-term care and nursing home care, based on U.S. and international models

REQUIRED TEXTS

Carlson, E. (2005). *20 common nursing home problems—and how to resolve them.* National Senior Citizens Law Center. Available for purchase from http://www.nsclc.org/publications/manuals/manual.2006-06-08.3692004924

Rantz, M. J., & Flesner, M. K. (2004). *Person centered care: A model for nursing homes.* Washington, DC: American Nurses Association with the University of Iowa College of Nursing.

Rantz, M., Popejoy, L., & Zwygart-Stauffacher, M. (2001). *The new nursing homes: A 20-minute way to find great long-term care.* Minneapolis, MN: Fairview Press.

REQUIREMENTS

All papers should be double spaced with decent margins, and all citations should be in APA style. You must give full credit to any sources used. Include a list of references with both papers. Provide the full citation with each reflection piece. Include references with the group presentation.

Quiz: Students will be quizzed on key terms and concepts.

Reflections on assigned readings: Record your reactions (1–2 pages typed) to eight class readings. Be prepared to discuss the readings and your reflections in class. Reflections should be organized around what information was new to you, and how this reading could relate to residents' quality-of-care or quality-of-life issues.

Group presentation: Groups of two to four students will work together to develop a twenty-minute PowerPoint presentation, which they will then deliver to the class. Each group should develop an outline of the presentation; this handout will be provided to all members of the class on the day of the presentation. Presentations should provide background on the issue, how the issue relates to quality of care and quality of life, and other contemporary controversies related to the issue. Each group must select a different topic. Possible topics include:

How much profit in for-profit nursing homes?

Feeding assistants

Oral health

Falls and restraints

Weight training

Staff criminal background checks

CPR in nursing homes

Hospice in nursing homes

Paper 1: Read *The New Nursing Homes: A 20-Minute Way to Find Great Long-Term Care.* Use the worksheet questions to compare and contrast two nursing homes, one in a rural area and one in an urban area. Call the administrator of each nursing home, and ask if you can visit for a school assignment. Also ask for permission to speak with/interview a director of nursing, social service director, activities director, or administrator. Use your own observations to complete the walk-through questions (chapter 2). Complete the staff questions (chapter 3) based on your interview of a staff member. Write a paper (9–11 pages) describing your experiences, and link your findings to at least four assigned readings. Include information you learned about the nursing home from the CMS Web site "Nursing Home Compare," and attach the findings to your paper in the appendix. The focus of the paper should be on quality of care and quality of life.

Paper 2: Write a paper (5–7 pages) discussing Rantz and Flesner's *Person Centered Care* in relation to these four concepts: resident rights, nurse aide roles and quality of care, financing of nursing home care, and nursing home regulations.

Class participation: Students will learn much from the experiences and insights of other students and are therefore expected to attend and participate in class. Attendance will be taken.

Graduate credit: Students receiving graduate credit for this course will be expected to complete the following additional assignment on a pass/fail basis: Write a paper discussing how one country's government—other than the

United States—pays for the long-term care needs of frail elders, both those living at home and in institutions. This paper should be eight to ten pages long.

COURSE OUTLINE

Session 1 Intro to course

Reading:

CDC. (2002). The national nursing home survey: 1999 summary. *Vital and Health Statistics,* Series 13, #152. DHHS, NCHS, CDC. Pages 1–5 only.

American Medical Directors Association. (n.d.). *Commonly used abbreviations, acronyms and terms in long term care.* Available at http://www.amda.com/tools/ltc_acronyms.cfm

Role of Nursing Homes in U.S. Long-Term Care System and Background: The Big Picture

Session 2 Historical context

Reading:

Holstein, M., & Cole, T R. (1996). The evolution of long-term care in America. In R. H. Binstock, L. E. Cluff, & O. von Mering (Eds.), *The future of long-term care: Social and policy issues* (pp. 19–47). Baltimore, MD: Johns Hopkins Press.

Kane, R. A. (1996). The evolution of the American nursing home. In H. Binstock, L. E. Cluff, & O. von Mering (Eds.), *The future of long-term care: Social and policy issues* (pp. 145–168). Baltimore, MD: Johns Hopkins University Press.

Lacey, D. (1999). The evolution of care: A 100-year history of institutionalization of people with Alzheimer's disease. *Journal of Gerontological Social Work, 31*(3/4), 101–131.

Session 3 Functional status (ADL, IADL)

Reading:

Cutler, D. M. (2001). Declining disability among the elderly. *Health Affairs, 20*(6), 11–27.

IADL and ADL scales

Lubitz, J., Liming, C., Kramarow, E., & Lentzer, H. (2003). Health, life expectancy, and health care spending among the elderly. *New England Journal of Medicine, 349*(11), 1048–1055. See table 2 and figures 1, 2, and 3.

Tripp-Reimer, T. (1997). Ethnicity, aging, and chronic illness. In E. A. Swanson & T. Tripp-Reimer (Eds.), *Advances in gerontological nursing: Chronic illness and the older adult* (pp. 112–135). New York: Springer.

Session 4 Who pays for care? Part 1

Reading:

Fact sheets. Available at http://ltc.georgetown.edu/papers.html

Spillman, B. C., & Lubitz, J. (2002). New estimates of lifetime nursing home use: Have patterns changed? *Medical Care, 40*(10), 965–975.

Session 5 Who pays for care? Part 2

Reading:

Feder, J., Komisar, H. L., & Niefeld, M. (2000). Long-term care in the United States: An overview. *Health Affairs, 19*(3), 40–56.

Rhoades, J. A., & Sommers, J. P. (2003). Trends in nursing home expenses, 1987 and 1996. *Health Care Financing Review, 25*(1), 99–114.

Session 6 OBRA federal regulations

Reading:

Burger, S. G., Fraser, V., Hunt, S., & Frank, B. (1996). Cornerstone of care: Residents' rights. In *Nursing homes: Getting good care there* (pp. 23–38). Washington, DC: National Citizens' Coalition for Nursing Home Reform.

Institute of Medicine. (2001). Information systems for monitoring quality. In *Improving the quality of long-term care* (pp. 110–134). Washington, DC: Author.

MDS form

Medicare. (n.d.). *Nursing home compare.* Available at http://www.medicare.gov/Nursing/Overview.asp

Turnham, H. *OBRA '87 Federal Nursing Home Reform Act: Summary.* Available at http://www.ltcombudsman.org/ombpublic/49_346_1023.cfm

Session 7 Quality

Reading:

Deutschman, M. (2001). Redefining quality and excellence in the nursing home culture. *Journal of Gerontological Nursing, 27*(8), 28–36.

International field test results of the observable indicators of nursing home care quality instrument. (2002). *International Nursing Review, 49,* 234–242.

Kane, R. A., Kling, K. C., Bershadsky, B., Kane, R. L., Giles, K., Degenholtz, H. B., et al. (2003). Quality of life measures for nursing home residents. *Journal of Gerontology: Medical Sciences, 58A*(3), 240–248.

Lawton, M. P. (2001). The physical environment of the person with Alzheimer's disease. *Aging and Mental Health, 5*(Suppl.), S56–S64.

Session 8 Nursing home field trip

Reading:

Nolan, M., & Tolson, D. (2000). Gerontological nursing 3: Valuing nursing homes and valuing staff. *British Journal of Nursing, 9*(3), 157–160.

Session 9 Quiz on main terms and concepts

The People in Nursing Homes

Session 10 Overview of staff

Reading:

American Medical Directors Association. *What is a medical director?* Available at http://www.amda.com/consumers/Medical Director.cfm

Birkett, D. P. (2001). The staff. In *Psychiatry in the nursing home* (2nd ed., pp. 53–68). New York: Haworth Press.

Bonifazi, W. L. (1999). A day in the life of a C.N.A. *Contemporary Long Term Care, 22*(5), 34–44.

Diamond, T. (1992). How do you make it on just one job? In *Making grey gold: Narratives of nursing home care* (pp. 35–52). Chicago: University of Chicago Press.

Student presentation: Feeding assistants

Session 11 Physical conditions: Dementia and delirium

Reading:

Espino, D. V., Mouton, C. P., Aguila, D. D., Parker, R. W., Lewis, R. M., & Miles, T. P. (2001). Mexican American elders with dementia in long term care. *Clinical Gerontologist, 23*(3/4), 83–96.

Fact sheet. Available at http://ihcrp.georgetown.edu/aging society/pdfs/alzheimers.pdf

Folstein Mini–Mental Assessment Exam

National Academy on an Aging Society. *Alzheimer's disease and dementia: A growing challenge.* Available at http://www.agingsociety.org/agingsociety/pdf/Alzheimers.pdf

Guest speaker: Social worker

Session 12 Depression and anxiety

Reading:

Geriatric Depression Scale

McInnis-Dittrich, K. (2005). Differential assessment and diagnosis of cognitive and emotional problems of elders. In *Social work with elders: A biopsychosocial approach to assessment and intervention* (2nd ed., pp. 116–150). Boston: Pearson, Allen and Bacon.

Session 13 Dehydration

Reading:

Kayser-Jones, J. (2002). Malnutrition, dehydration, and starvation in the midst of plenty: The political impact of qualitative inquiry. *Qualitative Health Research, 12*(10), 1391–1405.

Guest speaker: Director of nursing

Session 14 Film: *Confessions of a Dutiful Daughter*

Session 15 Psychosocial and spiritual issues

Reading:

Haberkost, M., Dellman-Jenkins, M., & Bennett, J. M. (1996). Importance of quality recreation activities for older adults residing in nursing homes: Considerations for gerontologists. *Educational Gerontology, 22,* 735–745.

Hartz, G. W., & Splain, D. M. (1997). Psychosocial needs of LTC residents. In *Psychosocial intervention in long-term care: An advanced guide* (pp. 11–28). New York: Haworth Press.

Koenig, H. G., Weiner, D. K., Peterson, B. L., Meador, K. G., & Keefe, F. J. (1997). Religious coping in the nursing home: A biopsychosocial model. *International Journal of Psychiatry in Medicine, 27*(4), 365–376.

Guest speaker: Chaplain

Session 16 Family members' perspectives

Reading:

Gladstone, J., & Wexler, E. (2000). A family perspective of family/staff interaction in long-term care. *Geriatric Nursing, 21*(1), 16–19.

Iwasiw, C., Goldenberg, D., Bol, N., & MacMaster, E. (2003). Resident and family perspectives: The first year in a long-term care facility. *Journal of Gerontological Nursing, 29*(1), 45–54.

Solomon, R. (1983). Serving families of the institutionalized aged: The four crises. In G. S. Getzel & M. J. Mellor (Eds.), *Gerontological social work practice in long-term care* (pp. 83–96). New York: Haworth Press.

Guest speaker: Family member

Session 17 Student presentations
Oral health
Falls and restraints

Session 18 Visit nursing home or work on papers
Start reading Rantz & Flesner

Session 19 Student presentations
Staff criminal background checks
Weight training

Session 20 Advance directives and medical decision making

Reading:

Forbes, S., Bern-Klug, M., & Gessert, C. (2000). End-of-life decision making for nursing home residents with dementia. *Journal of Nursing Scholarship, 32*(3), 251–258.

Kauffman, S. R. (1998). Intensive care, old age, and the problem of death in America. *The Gerontologist, 38*(6), 715–725.

Student presentation: CPR in nursing homes

Session 21 Death and dying (part 1)

Reading:

Bern-Klug, M., Gessert, C. E., Crenner, C. W., Buenaver, M., & Skirchak, D. (2004). "Getting everyone on the same page": Nursing home physicians' perspectives on end-of-life care. *Journal of Palliative Medicine, 7*(4), 533–544.

Wurzbach, M. E. (2002). End-of-life treatment decisions in long-term care. *Journal of Gerontological Nursing, 28*(6), 14–21.

Student presentation: Hospice in nursing homes

Session 22 Death and dying (part 2)
Paper 1 due

Reading:

Teno, J. M. (2004). Do-not-resuscitate orders and hospitalization of nursing home residents: Trumping, neglect, or shared decision-making at the eleventh hour? [Editorial]. *Journal of the American Geriatrics Society, 52,* 159–160.

Wilkinson, A. M., & Lynn, J. (2001). The end of life. In R. H. Binstock & L. K. George (Eds.), *Handbook of aging in the social sciences* (5th ed., pp. 444–461). San Diego, CA: Academic Press.

Session 23 Legal issues

Reading:

Carlson (2005)

National Citizen's Coalition on Nursing Home Reform. *Fact sheets: Abuse and neglect.* Available at http://www.nursinghomeaction.org/public/50_156_450.cfm

Guest speaker: Elder-law attorney

Innovations in Long-Term Care and International Long-Term Care

Session 24 Eden and Pioneer

Reading:

Fahey, C. J. (2003). Culture change in long-term care facilities: Changing the facility or changing the system? *Journal of Social Work in Long-Term Care, 2*(1/2), 35–51.

Thomas, W. H. (2003). Evolution of Eden. *Journal of Social Work in Long-Term Care, 2*(1/2), 141–157.

See "New language for a new culture." Available at http://www.pioneernetwork.net/stories-from-the-field/LanguageofCultureChange.php

Session 25 Film: *Eden Alternative*

Session 26 Person-centered care

Reading:

Rantz & Flesner

Session 27 More on person-centered care

Session 28 International approaches to long-term care

Reading:

Kane, R. A., Kane, R. L., & Ladd, R. C. (1998). International perspectives on long-term care. In *The heart of long-term care* (pp. 267–282). New York: Oxford University Press.

Course evaluation

Session 29 Nursing homes in 2040

Paper 2 due

BIBLIOGRAPHY

Allegre, A., Frank, B., & McIntosh, E. (1999). Hospice in the nursing home: A valuable collaboration. *Bioethics Forum, 15*(3), 7–12.

Beaulieu, E. M. (2002). *A guide for nursing home social workers.* New York: Springer.

Caplan, A. (1990). The morality of the mundane: Ethical issues arising in the daily lives of nursing home residents, In R. A. Kane & A. L. Caplan (Eds.), *Everyday ethics: Resolving dilemmas in nursing home life* (pp. 37–50). New York: Springer.

Finucane, T. E., & Harper, G. M. (1999). Attempting resuscitation in nursing homes: Policy considerations. *Journal of the American Geriatrics Society, 47,* 1261–1264.

Gass, T. E. (2004). *Nobody's home: Candid reflections of a nursing home aide.* Ithaca, NY: Cornell University Press.

Gubrium, J. E. (1975). *Living and dying in Murray Manor.* New York: St. Martin's Press.

Kane, R. A., & Caplan, A. L. (1990). Beyond the call of duty: A nurse's aide uses her judgment. In R. A. Kane & A. L. Caplan (Eds.), *Everyday ethics: Resolving dilemmas in nursing home life* (pp. 199–208). New York: Springer.

McGowin, D. F. (1993). *Living in the labyrinth: A personal journey through the maze of Alzheimer's*. New York: Bantam Doubleday Dell.

Mukamel, D. B., & Spector, W. D. (2003). Quality report cards and nursing home quality. *The Gerontologist, 43*(Special Issue 2), 58–66.

Ouslander, J. G., Osterweil, D., & Morley, J. (1991). *Medical care in the nursing home* (2nd ed.). New York: McGraw-Hill.

Powers, B. A. (2001). Ethnographic analysis of everyday ethics in the care of nursing home residents with dementia: A taxonomy. *Nursing Research, 50*(6), 332–339.

Rantz, M. J., Mehr, D. R., Popejoy, L., Zwygart-Stauffacher, M., Hicks, L. L., Grando, V., et al. (1998). Nursing home care quality: A multidimensional theoretical model. *Journal of Nursing Care Quality, 12*(3), 30–46.

Seaton, G. (2002). *The crisis in America's nursing homes: What are we doing wrong?* Republic of Ireland: Adverbage.

Tulloch, G. J. (1975). *A home is not a home: Life within a nursing home*. New York: Seabury Press.

Wiener, J. M. (2003). An assessment of strategies for improving quality of care in nursing homes. *The Gerontologist, 43*(Special Issue 2), 19–27.

30

When Mourning Is Complicated

Helen Harris

COURSE DESCRIPTION

This course will begin with a brief overview of a framework for understanding loss and grief and therapeutic interventions for the bereaved. The major focus of the course will then be on the circumstances that may produce complicated mourning; the assessment of complicated mourning; and micro, mezzo, and macro interventions with mourners and their support systems. The course will cover cultural and congregational responses to grief and loss.

OBJECTIVES

Upon completion of this course, students should be able to:

- Understand the dynamics and dimensions of grief and mourning following a loss and be able to normalize the experience for the bereaved
- Identify special types of losses with particular risk for complicated mourning
- Assess grief responses, including complicated mourning and risk factors for pathological responses
- Identify micro and mezzo treatment interventions for complicated mourning
- Identify macro interventions to better utilize community and congregational resources to meet the needs of the bereaved, including those with complex losses

REQUIRED TEXT

McCall, J. B. (2004). *Bereavement counseling: Pastoral care for complicated grieving*. Binghamton, NY: Haworth Press.

SUPPLEMENTAL TEXT

Rando, T. A. (1998). *Treatment of complicated mourning.* Champaign, IL: Research Press.

ASSIGNMENTS

All students must read McCall, chapters 1–5, prior to the first class session, and chapters 6–8 prior to the second class session.

Recommended reading: Rando, chapters 1–9, 12, 14.

Required reading log: Read the text and provide a one-page (type-written, single-spaced) annotation on the text. Include particular ideas you wish to remember and ways you can adapt what you have read to your professional practice. List key words at the end of the annotation.

Students will choose from the following assignments:

Complicated mourning group curriculum: Develop a six-to-eight-session curriculum for a grief support group for clients dealing with complicated mourning. Include information about group purpose, group admission process, group rules, and content/activities for the six to eight weeks.

Critical book review: Write a review of a book (3 pages minimum), preapproved by the professor, that deals grief, loss, and complicated mourning (may include congregational care of the bereaved).

Design your own assignment: Design a project that will assist you in achieving the learning objectives of this course. Your project must be approved by the professor. Some options are designing a curriculum for a complicated mourning training session in a church, writing a therapeutic song, creating an art project or a slide show that addresses complicated mourning, and videotaping interviews of parents who have lost a child or survivors of traumatic events that resulted in the death of loved ones.

Personal reaction papers: Write two pages describing an event, the emotional impact it had on you, and the learning that you experienced as a result. You may do one paper for each of the following topics.

- Personal reaction to an actual traumatic event, current or historical, involving loss and grief that is personal or societal in scope (e.g., loss of a parent, sudden loss of a loved one, the Mount Carmel tragedy, the bombing at Oklahoma City, national grief response to John Kennedy Jr.'s death, and response to the World Trade Center attack)
- Personal reaction to a created event (i.e., a film, song, book, poem, work of art) that involves death, loss, and complicated bereavement

- Personal reaction to one of the segments of class material or to a bereavement support group meeting that you attend

Paper describing church doctrinal positions and procedures for addressing the needs of the bereaved and their families: Write a paper (five pages minimum) that delineates the church or denominational position statement regarding needs and care of the bereaved and their families, the specific church ministries (formal and informal) to the bereaved and their families, and any training or instruction required by the church or available in the church for ministerial staff working with the bereaved and their families, particularly in the area of complicated mourning.

COURSE OUTLINE

Session 1	Normal grief, loss, and responses Reading: Chapters 1–2
Session 2	Complicated mourning assessment Reading: Chapters 3–5
Session 3	Complicated mourning intervention: Theory and treatment Reading: Chapters 6–7
Session 4	New beginnings: Micro, mezzo, and macro Reading: Chapter 8

BIBLIOGRAPHY

Bombeck, E. (1989). *I want to grow hair, I want to grow up, I want to go to Boise: Children surviving cancer.* New York: Harper and Row.

Burns, O. A. (1989). *Cold sassy tree.* New York: Dell.

Buscaglia, L. (1989). *The fall of Freddie the leaf.* New York: Holt, Rinehart and Winston.

Caplan, S., & Lang, G. (1989). *Grief's courageous journey.* Oakland, CA: New Harbinger Publications.

Connelly, R. J. (1992). *Last rights: Death and dying in Texas law and experience.* San Antonio, TX: Corona.

Cook, A. S., & Dworkin, D. S. (1992). *Helping the bereaved: Therapeutic interventions for children, adolescents, and adults.* New York: Basic Books.

Corr, C. A., Morgan, J. D., & Wass, H. (1992). *International work group on death, dying and bereavement: Statements on death, dying, and bereavement.* Ontario: International Work Group on Death, Dying and Bereavement, through King's College.

Corr, C. A., Nabe, C. M., & Corr, D. M. (1992). *Death and dying, life and living.* Belmont, CA: Wadsworth.

DeSpelder, L. A., & Srickland, A. L. (1995). *The path ahead: Readings in death and dying.* Mountain View, CA: Mayfield.

Dickinson, G. E., & Leming, M. R. (1994). *Dying, death, and bereavement* (2nd ed.). Guilford, CT: Dushkin.

Dietz, S. D., & Hicks, M. J. P. (1989). *Take these broken wings and learn to fly: The AIDS support book for patients, family and friends*. Tucson, AZ: Harbinger House.

Doka, K. J. (Ed.). (1995). *Children mourning, mourning children*. Washington, DC: Hospice Foundation of America.

Doka, K. J. (Ed.). (1996). *Living with grief after sudden loss: Suicide, homicide, accident, heart attack, stroke*. Washington, DC: Hospice Foundation of America.

Doka, K. J. (Ed.). (1997). *Living with grief: When illness is prolonged*. Washington, DC: Hospice Foundation of America.

Doka, K. J. (Ed.). (1998). *Living with grief: Who we are, how we grieve*. Washington, DC:. Hospice Foundation of America.

Doka, K. J. (Ed.). (2000). *Living with grief: Children, adolescents and loss*. Washington, DC: Hospice Foundation of America.

Epstein, H. (1979). *Children of the Holocaust: Conversations with sons and daughters of survivors*. New York: G. P. Putnam's Sons.

Furth, G. M. (1988). *The secret world of drawings: Healing through art*. Boston: Sigo Press.

Gaes, J. (1987). *My book for kids with cansur: A child's autobiography of hope*. Aberdeen, SD: Melius and Peterson.

Gallo, J., Reichel, W., & Andersen, L. (1988). *Handbook of geriatric assessment*. Rockville, MD: Aspen.

Gersie, A. (1991). *Storymaking in bereavement: Dragons fight in the meadow*. Bristol, PN: Jessica Kingsley.

Goldman, L. (1996). *Breaking the silence: A guide to help children with complicated grief—suicide, homicide, aids, violence, and abuse*. Washington, DC: Taylor and Francis.

Grollman, E. A. (1987). *Time remembered: A journal for survivors*. Boston: Beacon Press.

Grollman, E. A. (Ed.). (1995). *Bereaved children and teens*. Boston: Beacon Press.

Grollman, E. A. (1995). *Living when a loved one has died*. Boston: Beacon Press.

Gruetzner, H. (1992). *Alzheimer's: A caregiver's guide and sourcebook*. New York: John Wiley and Sons.

Jensen, M. (1982). *First we have coffee*. San Bernardino, CA: Here's Life Publishers.

Kastenbaum, R. J. (1998). *Death, society, and human experience* (6th ed.). Boston: Allyn and Bacon.

Kirschling, J. M. (Ed.). (1990). *Family-based palliative care*. New York: Haworth Press.

Kübler-Ross, E. (1975). *Death: The final stage of growth*. Englewood Cliffs, NJ: Prentice-Hall.

Kübler-Ross, E. (1997). *The wheel of life: A memoir of living and dying*. New York: Scribner.

Lancaster, M. (1983). *Hang tough*. New York: Paulist Press.

Larson, D. G. (1993). *The helper's journey: Working with people facing grief, loss, and life-threatening illness*. Champaign, IL: Research Press.

McCue, K. (1994). *How to help children through a parent's serious illness*. New York: St. Martin's Press.

Miller, J. E. (1992). *How will I get through the holidays? 12 ideas for those whose loved one has died*. Fort Wayne, IN: Willowgreen Productions.

Miller, J. E. (1997). *Helping the bereaved celebrate the holidays: A sourcebook for planning instructional and remembrance events.* Fort Wayne, IN: Willowgreen Productions.

Moffatt, B. C. (1988). *Gifts for the living: Conversations with caregivers on death and dying.* Santa Monica, CA: IBS Press.

Paulus, T. (1972). *Hope for the flowers.* New York: Paulist Press.

Pojman, L. P. (1993). *Life and death: A reader in moral problems.* Sudbury, MA: Jones and Bartlett.

Rando, T. A. (1986). *Loss and anticipatory grief.* Lexington, MA: Lexington Books.

Rollin, B. (1985). *Last wish.* New York: Linden Press.

Siegel, B. S. (1986). *Love, medicine and miracles.* New York: Harper and Row.

Smith, S. C., & Pennells, M. (Eds.). (1995). *Interventions with bereaved children.* Bristol, PN: Jessica Kingsley.

Spring, B., & Larson, E. (1988). *Euthanasia: Spiritual, medical and legal issues in terminal health care.* Portland, OR: Multnomah Press.

Temes, R. (1977). *Living with an empty chair.* New York: Irvington.

Traisman, E. S. (1992). *Fire in my heart, ice in my veins: A journal for teenagers experiencing a loss.* Burnsville, NC: Centering Corporation.

Turk, D. C., & Feldman, C. S. (1992). *Noninvasive approaches to pain management in the terminally ill.* New York: Haworth Press.

Wass, H., & Neimeyer, R. A. (1995). *Dying: Facing the facts.* Washington, DC: Taylor and Francis.

Wiesel, E. (1961). *Dawn.* Chicago: Avon Bard Books.

Wolfelt, A. D. (1992). *Sarah's journey: One child's experience with the death of her father.* Fort Collins, CO: Center for Loss and Life Transition.

Wolfelt, A. D. (1994). *Healing the bereaved child: Grief gardening, growth through grief and other touchstones for caregivers.* Fort Collins, CO: Companion Press.

Wolterstorff, N. (1987). *Lament for a son.* Grand Rapids, MI: William B. Eerdmans.

Worden, J. W. (1982). *Grief counseling and grief therapy: A handbook for the mental health practitioner* (1st ed.). New York: Springer.

31

Social Work in Pediatric Palliative and End-of-Life Care

Barbara Jones

COURSE DESCRIPTION

This advanced practice course is designed to provide a framework for clinical practice with children and families who are facing life-threatening conditions, end of life, and bereavement. This course will enhance the knowledge base of clinical social work students and will be useful to students interested in learning about the medical, psychosocial, and spiritual needs of children and their families as they approach the end of life. Utilizing a stance of respect, cultural humility, and reflexive practice, students will engage in a learning environment that is designed to empower them and give them skills to empower children and families facing the end of life.

The topics for the course are the results of a mixed-methodology study with pediatric oncology social workers practicing palliative and end-of-life care. The main topics for the educational experience are based on the empirical findings of this study. There is a strong emphasis on reflective and reflexive practice and self-care throughout the course. The theoretical frameworks that guide the course are family centered, empowerment, strengths based, multicultural, ethical, and ethnographic. The social work student is expected to appreciate children with life-threatening conditions and their families as important teachers in their unique needs.

The student will be asked to adopt a stance of openness and compassion that acknowledges the primacy of the experience of the child/family, an ethical duty to advocate for the child's/family's needs, cultural humility and awareness, reflexive practice, and willingness to collaborate with other professionals in education, research, and practice.

The learning environment will include lecture, guest speakers, film, music, poetry, art, field trips, contemplation, and group exercises in an attempt to deliver an intellectual and meaningful experience.

COURSE OBJECTIVES

By the end of this course, students will be able to:

- Understand the impact of life-threatening conditions on children and families
- Articulate their personal relationships to illness, death, and loss and understand the significance of this relationship to the helping process
- Understand the common psychosocial and spiritual challenges faced by children and family members coping with life-threatening illness and death
- Demonstrate an understanding of the cultural factors at work in the clinical interface with children and families
- Develop reflective awareness of the knowledge brought by clinicians and by children and their families to the clinical encounter
- Demonstrate familiarity with literature related to palliative and bereavement care with children and families
- Identify social and cultural obstacles to the provision of optimal clinical services to children and families
- Demonstrate an understanding of clinical interventions helpful to children and families coping with illness, death, and bereavement

COURSE REQUIREMENTS

Regular attendance is essential; students should be prepared to discuss readings and relevant personal and professional experience during class. Engagement in class discussion will be considered in the assessment process.

In addition, students will be expected to complete written assignments that will explore their personal loss history and their reflections on this work and a final research paper.

ASSIGNMENTS AND GRADING

Assignment	Weight
Personal loss history paper	20%
Journal	20%
Attendance and participation	10%
Agency visit and written reflection	20%
Final paper on pediatric palliative care	30%

REQUIRED TEXT

Institute of Medicine. (2003). *When children die: Improving palliative and end-of-life care for children and their families* (M. J. Field & R. E. Behrman, Eds.). Washington, DC: National Academy Press.

COURSE OUTLINE

Session 1 Introduction to pediatric palliative care

Reading:
Institute of Medicine, chapters 1 and 2

American Academy of Pediatrics. (2000). Palliative care for children. *Pediatrics, 106,*(2), 351–357. Available at http://www.aap.org/policy/re0007.html

Browning, D. (2004). Fragments of love: Explorations in the ethnography of suffering and professional caregiving. In J. Berzoff & P. Silverman (Eds.), *Living with dying: A handbook for end-of-life care healthcare practitioners* (pp. 21–42). New York: Columbia University Press.

Hilden, J. M., Himelstein, B. P., Freyer, D. R., Friebert, S., & Kane, J. R. (2001). End-of-life care: Special issues in pediatric oncology. In K. Foley & H. Gelband (Eds.), *Improving palliative care for cancer* (pp. 161–198). Washington, DC: National Academy Press.

Stillion, J., & Papadatou, D. (2002). Suffer the children: An examination of psychosocial issues in children and adolescents with terminal illness. *American Behavioral Scientist, 46*(2), 299–315.

Session 2 The unique needs of children with life-threatening conditions

Reading:
Institute of Medicine, chapter 3

Attig, T. (1996). Beyond pain: The existential suffering of children. *Journal of Palliative Care, 12*(3), 20–23.

Gibbons, M. B. (2001). Psychosocial aspects of serious illness in childhood and adolescence: Curse or challenge? In A. Armstrong-Dailey & S. Zarbock (Eds.), *Hospice care for children* (2nd ed., pp. 49–67). New York: Oxford University Press.

Jones, B., & Weisenfluh, S. (2003). Pediatric palliative and end-of-life care: Developmental and spiritual issues of dying children. *Smith College Studies in Social Work. Special Issue on End-of-Life Care, 73*(3), 421–442.

Noll, R. B., Gartstein, M. A., Vannatta, K., Correll, J., Bukowski, W. M., & Davies, W. H. (1999). Social, emotional, and behavioral functioning of children with cancer. *Pediatrics, 103*(1) 71–78.

Session 3 The unique needs of families and siblings

Reading:
Institute of Medicine, chapter 4

Bengston, V. L. (2001). Beyond the nuclear family: The increasing importance of multigenerational bonds. *Journal of Marriage and Family Therapy, 63,* 116.

Bluebond-Langner, M. (1995). Worlds of dying children and their well siblings. In K. J. Doka (Ed.), *Children mourning, mourning children* (pp. 115–130). Washington, DC: Hospice Foundation of America.

Contro, N., Larson, J., Scofield, S., Sourkes, B., & Cohen, H. J. (2002). Family perspectives on the quality of pediatric palliative care. *Archives of Pediatrics and Adolescent Medicine, 156*(1), 14–19.

Davies, B. (1991). Long-term outcome of adolescent sibling bereavement. *Journal of Adolescent Research, 6,* 83–96.

Gibbons, M. (1992). A child dies, a child survives: The impact of sibling loss. *Journal of Pediatric Care, 6,* 65–72.

Meyer, E., Burns, J. P., Griffith, J. L., & Truoq, R. D. (2002). Parental perspectives on end-of-life care in the pediatric intensive care unit. *Critical Care Medicine, 30*(1), 226–231.

Teno, J. M., Clarridge, B. R., Casey, V., Welch, L. C., Wetle, T., Shield, R., et al. (2004). Family perspectives on end-of-life care at the last place of care. *Journal of American Medical Association, 291*(1), 88–93.

Session 4 Developmentally appropriate assessment and intervention with children

Reading:

Boyd-Webb, N. (2003). Play and expressive therapies to help bereaved children: Individual, family and group treatment. *Smith College Studies in Social Work. Special Issue on End-of-Life Care, 73*(3), 403–420.

Eng, B. (1999). Puppets: Bridging the communication gap between caregivers and children about death and dying. In S. Bertman (Ed.), *Grief and the healing arts: Creativity as therapy* (pp. 127–138). Amityville, NY: Baywood.

Faulkner, K. W. (1993). Children's understanding of death. In A. Armstrong-Dailey & S. Z. Goltzer (Eds.), *Hospice care for children* (pp. 9–21). New York: Oxford University Press.

Piaget, J. (2001). *The child's conception of physical causality.* New Brunswick, NJ: Transaction Publishers.

Sourkes, B. (1999). Art techniques for children with cancer. In S. Bertman (Ed.), *Grief and the healing arts: Creativity as therapy* (pp. 119–125). Amityville, NY: Baywood.

Sourkes, B. (2000). Psychotherapy with the dying child. In H. M. Chechinov & W. Breibart (Eds.), *Handbook of psychiatry in palliative medicine* (pp. 265–272). Oxford: Oxford University Press.

Session 5 The role of social work in pediatric palliative care and interdisciplinary teams

Reading:

Institute of Medicine, chapters 5 and 6.

Abramson, J., & Mizrahi, T. (1996). When social workers and physicians collaborate: Positive and negative interdisciplinary experiences. *Social Work, 41*(3), 270–281.

Beck, A. (2000). Communication between professions: Doctors are from Mars, social workers are from Venus. *Journal of Palliative Medicine, 3*(2), 221–222.

Christ, G. C., & Sormanti, M. (1999). Advancing social work practice in end-of-life care. *Social Work in Health Care, 30*(2), 81–99.

Clark, E. J. (2004). The future of social work in end-of-life care: A call to action. In J. Berzoff & P. Silverman (Eds.), *Living with dying: A handbook for end-of-life healthcare practitioners* (pp. 838–847). New York: Columbia University Press.

Cummings, I. (1998). The interdisciplinary team. In D. Doyle, G. W. C. Hanks, & N. MacDonald (Eds.), *Oxford textbook of palliative medicine* (2nd ed., pp. 19–30). Oxford: Oxford University Press.

Hobart, K. R. (2001). Death and dying and the social work role. *Journal of Gerontological Social Work, 36*(3/4), 181–192.

Small, N. (2001). Social work and palliative care. *British Journal of Social Work, 31,* 961–971.

Session 6 Counseling, companioning, and presence

Reading:

Chochinov, H. M. (2003). Thinking outside the box: Depression, hope and meaning at the end of life. *Journal of Palliative Medicine, 6*(6), 973–978.

Frank, A. W. (1998). Just listening: Narrative and deep illness. *Families, Systems, and Health, 16*(3), 197–216.

Sellick, M., Delaney, R., & Brownlee, K. (2002). The deconstruction of professional knowledge: Accountability without authority. *Families in Society: The Journal of Contemporary Human Services, 83*(5/6), 493–498.

Session 7 Advocacy, communication, and coordination

Reading:

Ambuel, B.(2000). Conducting a family conference. *Principles and Practice of Supportive Oncology, 3*(3) 1–12.

Doka, K. J. (1995). Talking to children about illness. In K. J. Doka (Ed.), *Children mourning: Mourning children* (pp. 31–40). Washington, DC: Hospice Foundation of America.

Dube, C. E., LaMonica, A., Boyle, W., Fuller, B., & Burkholder, G. J. (2003). Self-assessment of communication skills preparedness: Adult versus pediatric skills. *Ambulatory Pediatrics, 3*(3), 137–141.

Jankovic, M., Loiacono, N. B., Spinetta, J. J., Riva, L., Conter, V., & Masera, G. (1994). Telling young children with leukemia their diagnosis: The flower garden as analogy. *Pediatric Hematology and Oncology, 11,* 75–81.

Young, B., Dixon-Woods, M., Windridge, K. C., & Henry, D. (2003). Managing communication with young people who have a potentially life-threatening chronic illness: A qualitative study of patients and parents. *British Medical Journal, 326,* 305–310.

Session 8 Culture, ethnicity, and spirituality

Reading:

Institute of Medicine, Appendix C

Braun, K. L., Pietsch, J. H., & Blanchette, P. (Eds.). (1999). *Cultural issues in end-of-life decision making*. Thousand Oaks, CA: Sage.

Cosh, R. (1995). Spiritual care of the dying. In I. B. Corless, B. B. Germino & M. A. Pittman (Eds.), *Dying, death, and bereavement: A challenge for living* (pp. 131–144). Boston: Jones and Bartlett.

Koenig, B., & Gates-Williams, J. (1995). Understanding cultural differences in caring for dying patients. *Western Journal of Medicine, 163*(3), 244–249.

Laird, J. (1998). Theorizing culture: Narrative ideas and practice principles. In M. McGoldrick (Ed.), *Re-visioning family therapy: Race, culture, and gender in clinical practice* (pp. 20–36). New York: Guilford Press.

Parker, O. D. (2003). Social work and spiritual counseling. *Journal of Palliative Medicine, 6*(6), 919–925.

Parkes, C. M. (1997). Attachments and losses in cross-cultural perspective. In C. M. Parkes, P. Laungani, & B. Young (Eds.), *Death and bereavement across cultures* (pp. 233–243). New York: Routledge.

Session 9 Pain and symptom management

Reading:

Altilio, T. (2004). Pain and symptom management: An essential role for social work. In J. Berzoff & P. Silverman (Eds.), *Living with dying: A handbook for end-of-life care healthcare practitioners* (pp. 380–408). New York: Columbia University Press.

Franck, L. S., Greenburg, C. S., & Steven, B. (2000). Pain assessment in infants and children. *Pediatric Clinics of North America, 47*(3), 487–512.

Kuttner, L. (1996). How to relieve pain. In *A child in pain: How to help, what to do* (pp. 76–149). Point Roberts, WA: Hartley and Marks.

Mendenhall, M. (2003). Psychosocial aspects of pain management: A conceptual framework for social workers on pain management teams. *Social Work in Health Care, 36*(4), 35–51.

Wolfe, J., Grier, H. E., Klar, N., Levin, S. B., Ellenbogen, J. M., Salem-Schatz, S., et al. (2000). Symptoms and suffering at the end of life in children with cancer. *New England Journal of Medicine, 3*(5), 326–348.

Session 10 Ethics and ethical decision making

Reading:

Institute of Medicine, chapter 8

Browning, D. (2003). To show our humanness: Relational and communicative competence in pediatric palliative care. *Bioethics Forum, 18*(3/4), 23–28.

Chochinov, H. M. (2002). Dignity-conserving care: A new model for palliative care. *Journal of the American Medical Association, 287*(17), 2253–2260.

Csikai, E., Roth, S., & Moore, C. D. (2004). Ethical problems faced in end-of-life decision making by oncology social workers and the need for practice guidelines. *Journal of Psychosocial Oncology, 22*(1), 1–18.

Foster, L. W., & McLellan, L. J. (2002). Translating psychosocial insight into ethical discussions supportive of families in end-of-life decision-making. *Social Work in Health Care, 35*(3), 37–51.

Sullivan, M. D. (2002). The illusion of patient choice in end-of-life decisions. *American Journal of Geriatric Psychiatry, 10,* 365–372.

Session 11 Bereavement

Reading:

Institute of Medicine, Appendix E

Barrett, R. K. (1998). Sociocultural considerations for working with blacks experiencing loss and grief. In K. Doka & J. Davidson (Eds.), *Living with grief: Who we are, how we grieve* (pp. 83–96). Washington, DC: Hospice Foundation of America.

Fleming, S., & Balmer, L. (1991). Group intervention with bereaved children. In D. Papadatou & C. Papadatou (Eds.),

Children and death (pp. 105–124). Washington, DC: Hemisphere Publishing.

Klass, D. (2000). Solace and immortality: Bereaved parents' continuing bond with their children. *Death Studies, 17*(4), 343–368.

Neimeyer, R., Prigerson, H., & Davies, B. (2002). Mourning and meaning. *American Behavioral Scientist, 46*(2), 235–251.

Wilder, R. E. (1998). Sexual orientation and grief. In K. Doka & J. Davidson (Eds.), *Living with grief: Who we are, how we grieve* (pp. 199–206). Washington, DC: Hospice Foundation of America.

Session 12 Self-care: From the start

Reading:

Barnard, D. (1995). The promise of intimacy and the fear of our own undoing. *Journal of Palliative Care, 11*(4), 22–26.

Calhoun, L. G., & Tedeschi, R. G. (2001). Posttraumatic growth: The positive lessons of loss. In R. A. Neimeyer (Ed.), *Meaning reconstruction and the experience of loss* (pp. 157–172). Washington, DC: American Psychological Association.

Foster, Z., & Davidson, K. (1995). Satisfactions and stresses for the social worker. In I. B. Corless, B. B. Germino, & M. A. Pittman (Eds.), *Dying, death, and bereavement: A challenge for living* (pp. 131–144). Boston: Jones and Bartlett.

Katz, R., & Genevay, B. (2002). Our patients, our families, ourselves: The impact of the professional's emotional responses in end-of-life care. *American Behavioral Scientist, 46,* 327–339.

Papadatou, D. (2000). A proposed model of health care providers' grieving process. *Omega: Journal of Death and Dying, 41,* 59–77.

Webster, J., & Kristjanson, L. (2002). "But isn't it depressing?" The vitality of palliative care. *Journal of Palliative Care, 18*(1), 15–24.

ADDITIONAL RESOURCES FOR THE INSTRUCTOR

The Initiative for Pediatric Palliative Care has developed a six-module interdisciplinary training program, which is available free of charge at www.ippcweb.org. The downloadable modules are:

- Engaging with Children and Families
- Relieving Pain and Other Symptoms
- Analyzing Ethical Challenges in Pediatric End-of-Life Decision Making

- Responding to Suffering and Bereavement
- Improving Communication and Strengthening Relationships
- Establishing Continuity of Care

In addition to printed materials and classroom activities, there is a series of films available for each module that can be ordered through the Web site.

32

End-of-Life Decision Making

Susan Hedlund and Pamela Miller

COURSE DESCRIPTION

This course covers a broad range of topics related to social work and end-of-life care, including cultural and spiritual dimensions at end of life, pain and symptom management, end-of-life planning, hospice and palliative care, practice theory, ethical implications, policy and practice, team work, history, and resources. The course emphasizes the contributions of social work to end-of-life care within the context of our current political, cultural, and economic circumstances.

LEARNING OBJECTIVES

Upon completion of this course, students will be able to:

- Connect the history of the development of end-of-life care to the evolution of medical care in the United States from a policy/practice perspective
- Recognize practice innovations in palliative care and hospice
- Understand the role of social work in pain and symptom management and the contribution of a multidisciplinary team approach
- Discuss the need for planning at end of life through the use of advance directives and physician orders for life-sustaining treatment
- Explore the cultural and spiritual dimensions at end of life and the meaning and experience of suffering
- Utilize local, national, and online resources
- Identify the ethical challenges at end of life
- Demonstrate knowledge of social work theory and clinical interventions at the end of life

POPULATIONS AT RISK

Populations at risk are those who are intentionally and unintentionally discriminated against because of their possession of one or more attributes that are not valued by dominant society. Vulnerable persons are at increased risk of social isolation and economic disadvantage and its consequences because of the pervasive effects of structural inequality and their lack of access to power. People of color and ethnic diversity are represented in class readings, discussion, and case materials. Vulnerability secondary to poverty, sex, age, physical ability, and sexual orientation is a general concern.

REQUIRED TEXTS

Berzoff, J., & Silverman, P. R. (Eds.). (2004). *Living with dying*. New York: Columbia University Press.

Csikai, E. L., & Chaitin, E. (2006). *Ethics in end-of-life decisions in social work practice*. Chicago: Lyceum Books.

ASSIGNMENTS AND GRADING

You will develop a tabletop display that will be presented at our last class meeting. This meeting will take the form of an end-of-life conference at which the instructor and students will have the chance to view all students' work.

Grades will be based on the following criteria:

To receive an A, you must:

- Complete your own advance directives
- Complete the Web-based course from NASW, Understanding End of Life Care: The Social Worker's Role (available at http://www.naswwebed.org), and have certificate of completion on poster presentation
- Develop an annotated bibliography with eight references regarding an end-of-life issue
- Interview someone knowledgeable about end-of-life care and write a story about his or her perspectives (the person can be a health-care professional, patient, family member, or volunteer)

To receive a B, you must:

- Complete your own advance directives
- Develop an annotated bibliography with five references regarding an end-of-life issue
- Interview someone knowledgeable about end-of-life care and write a story about his or her perspectives (the person can be a health-care professional, patient, family member, or volunteer)
- Identify and describe three national resources regarding end-of-life care

To receive a B–, you must:

- Complete your own advance directives
- Develop an annotated bibliography with four references regarding an end-of-life issue
- Interview someone knowledgeable about end-of-life care and write a story about his or her perspectives (the person can be a health-care professional, patient, family member, or volunteer)

Your advance directive will not be opened or read. The idea behind this assignment is for you to consider the document and engage in discussions concerning it.

COURSE OUTLINE

Session 1 Course overview
Introductions
History of end-of-life care
Medical and social factors in end of life
Theory and practice

Session 2 National Association of Social Worker's Standards for Social Work in Palliative and End-of-Life Care
Advance directives and planning
Physician orders for life-sustaining treatment
Reading: Csikai & Chaitin, pp. 241–249, and chapters 3 and 5

Session 3 Spiritual, cultural, religious, and social diversity
Multicultural framework
Gays and lesbians
Marginalization
Disability
Reading: Csikai & Chaitin, chapter 2; Berzoff & Silverman, chapters 22–25

Session 4 Pediatric end-of-life care
Grief work
Reading: Handout on pediatrics and families
Guest speaker: Pediatric hemotology/oncology social worker

Session 5 Hospice and palliative care
Funeral options/conflicts
Reading: Csikai & Chaitin, chapter 4; check out http://www.nhpco.org

Session 6 Innovations in end-of-life care
Music thanatology
Guest speaker: Music thanatologist

Session 7	Pain and symptom management at the end of life: Working in teams Reading: Chapter 1, review chapters 3 and 8 Guest speaker
Session 8	Ethics at end of life Oregon's Death with Dignity Act Peruse the eighth-year report at http://www.oregon.gov/DHS/ph/pas/index.shtml Reading: Csikai & Chaitin, chapter 7; review chapters 2 and 3
Session 9	Guest speaker Work on poster presentation
Session 10	End-of-life poster session

33

Clinical Practice with Individuals and Families Coping with Life-Threatening Illness

Mary Sormanti

COURSE DESCRIPTION

This course is designed to provide a framework for clinical practice with individuals and families who are coping with a life-threatening illness. The course will enhance the skills and knowledge base of clinical practice students and may be particularly useful to students concentrating in the health, mental health, and disabilities or family and children's services fields of practice. Life-threatening illness is surrounded by a complex set of issues that will be addressed throughout the course. These include medical treatment choices, sociocultural forces that shape care provision and coping, multicultural perspectives on illness and death, psychosocial challenges and tasks associated with developmental stages, countertransference, and secondary stresses connected with this type of work. Social work skills vital in health-care practice will be examined, including biopsychosocial assessment, interventions such as discharge planning, case management, advocacy and outreach, interdisciplinary collaboration, crisis intervention, grief and bereavement therapy, and psychoeducation. As the health-care environment is rapidly changing, values and ethics in clinical practice will also be discussed.

COURSE OBJECTIVES

By the end of this course students will:

- Understand the impact of life-threatening illness on the individual and the entire family system

- Be able to articulate their own personal and culturally based beliefs about illness and evaluate the impact these have on the helping process
- Understand the common psychosocial challenges, adaptive tasks, and issues that clients at different developmental stages often face when coping with life-threatening illness
- Be familiar with social science, health, and mental health literature related to the psychosocial issues of life-threatening illness
- Understand the meaning and significance of different culturally based forms of client belief systems and coping mechanisms during the illness process
- Be able to identify critical organizational and environmental factors that affect clients' abilities to cope with life-threatening illness, including oppression, paternalism, poverty, and managed care
- Be able to demonstrate an understanding of social work interventions with empirical evidence of effectiveness in assisting clients coping with life-threatening illness

COURSE REQUIREMENTS

In an advanced practice class, professional dialogue and reflection are paramount. Accordingly, regular and timely attendance at each class is essential. In addition, students are expected to complete all reading assignments for each class and be prepared to draw from these and related fieldwork experiences during class discussions. An assessment of class participation will be incorporated into the student's final grade. Several written assignments are also required.

In this course students will write an illness history paper (due week #2) and a final paper (due week #7). The illness history assignment encourages the student to reflect upon his or her own experiences with illness and how these may affect his or her clinical work. The final paper provides students with an opportunity to critically apply what they have learned from class materials (i.e., readings, films, discussions) to a specific case from their fieldwork. Those students who do not have relevant fieldwork experience will be allowed to use fictional or nonfictional case material from books or films pending approval of the instructor.

COURSE OUTLINE

Session 1 Overview of clinical practice issues in life-threatening illness
Risk and protective factors over the life course
Social work role in a host setting and on multidisciplinary teams

Common stresses and rewards of the work
Skill development focus: Addressing death anxiety, self-awareness, and self-care

Required reading:
Crawley, L. M. (2005). Racial, cultural, and ethnic factors influencing end-of-life care. *Journal of Palliative Medicine, 8*(Suppl.), S58–69.
Dane, B., & Chachkes, E. (2001). The cost of caring for patients with an illness: Contagion to the social worker. *Social Work in Health Care, 33*(2), 31–51.

Session 2 The illness trajectory: Coping with diagnosis
Psychosocial challenges
Engagement and assessment issues
Skill development focus: Deep listening, crisis intervention, exploration of difficult topics
Illness history paper due

Required reading:
Frank, A. W. (1998). Just listening: Narrative and deep illness. *Families, Systems, and Health, 16*(3), 197–216.
Levenson, J. L. (2006). Psychiatric issues in oncology. *Primary Psychiatry, 13*(9), 31–34.
Nepo, M. (1997). God, self, and medicine. In J. Young-Mason (Ed.), *The patient's voice: Experiences of illness* (pp. 133–141). Philadelphia: F. A. Davis.
Spira, M., & Kenemore, E. (2002). Cancer as life transition: A relational approach to cancer wellness in women. *Clinical Social Work Journal, 30*(2), 173–186.

Session 3 The illness experience: Coping with treatment (part 1)
Psychosocial challenges for individuals and families
Skill development focus: Anxiety and pain management, supporting relational shifts, facilitating stabilization

Required reading:
Gawande, A. (1999, October 4). Whose body is it anyway? *New Yorker,* pp. 84–91.
Kagawa-Singer, M., & Blackhall, L. J. (2001). Negotiating cross-cultural issues at the end of life: "You got to go where he lives." *Journal of the American Medical Association, 286*(23), 2993–3001.
Macurdy, A. H. (1997). Mastery of life. In J. Young-Mason (Ed.), *The patient's voice: Experiences of illness* (pp. 9–15). Philadelphia: F. A. Davis.

Rolland, J. S. (2005). Chronic illness and the family life cycle. In B. Carter & M. McGoldrick (Eds.), *The expanded family life cycle: Individual, family, and social perspectives* (3rd ed., pp. 492–511). Boston: Allyn and Bacon.

Session 4 The illness experience: Coping with treatment (part 2)
Successful intervention strategies
Skill development focus: Co-creation of meaning and understanding; facilitation of family conferences

Required reading:

Altilio, T. (2004). Pain and symptom management: An essential role for social work. In J. Berzoff & P. Silverman (Eds.), *Living with dying: A handbook for healthcare practitioners* (pp. 380–408). New York: Columbia University Press.

Boyle, D. K., Miller, P. A., & Forbes-Thompson, S. A. (2005). Communication and end-of-life care in the intensive care unit: Patient, family, and clinician outcomes. *Critical Care Nursing Quarterly, 28*(4), 302–316.

Johnson, G., Kent, G., & Leather, J. (2005). Strengthening the parent-child relationship: A review of family interventions and their use in medical settings. *Child: Care, Health & Development, 31*(1), 25–32.

Recommended reading:

Simpson, E. (1997). The challenge. In J. Young-Mason (Ed.), *The patient's voice: Experiences of illness* (pp. 41–46). Philadelphia: F.A. Davis.

Simpson, G. (1997). Struggling. In J. Young-Mason (Ed.), *The patient's voice: Experiences of illness* (pp. 35–38). Philadelphia: F.A. Davis.

Session 5 The illness experience: Coping with impending death (part 1)
Psychosocial challenges faced by individuals and families
Ethical dilemmas
Skill development focus: Exploring values and priorities; anticipatory grief

Required reading:

Coyle, N. (2006). The hard work of living in the face of death. *Journal of Pain and Symptom Management, 32*(3), 266–274.

O'Donnell, P. (2004). Ethical issues in end-of-life care: Social work facilitation and proactive intervention. In J. Berzoff & P. Silverman (Eds.), *Living with dying: A handbook for healthcare practitioners* (pp. 171–187). New York: Columbia University Press.

Zilberfein, F., & Hurwitz, E. (2004). Clinical social work practice at the end of life. In J. Berzoff & P. Silverman (Eds.), *Living with dying: A handbook for healthcare practitioners* (pp. 297–317). New York: Columbia University Press.

Session 6 The illness experience: Coping with impending death (part 2)
Psychosocial challenges faced by individuals and families
Skill development focus: Exploring values and priorities

Required reading:

Carroll, R. (2005). Finding the words to say it: The healing power of poetry. *Evidence-Based Complementary and Alternative Medicine, 2*(2), 161–172.

Hinds, P. S., Schum, L., Baker, J. N., & Wolfe, J. (2005). Key factors affecting dying children and their families. *Journal of Palliative Medicine, 8*(S1), S70–S78.

Hood, A. (1999, Winter). In search of miracles. *Doubletake,* 62–69.

Session 7 Bereavement: Interventions with survivors
Overview of the natural bereavement process
Skill development focus: Differentiating normal from complicated grief
Final paper due

Required reading:

Dane, B. (2002). A brief treatment approach to bereavement. In B. Dane, C. Tosone, & A. Wolson (Eds.), *Doing more with less: Using long-term skills in short-term treatment* (pp. 405–432). Northvale, NJ: J. Aronson.

Shapiro, E. R. (1996). Family bereavement and cultural diversity: A social developmental perspective. *Family Process, 35*(3), 313–332.

Silverman, P.R. (2004). Bereavement: A time of transition and changing relationships. In J. Berzoff & P. Silverman (Eds.), *Living with dying: A handbook for healthcare practitioners* (pp. 226–241). New York: Columbia University Press.

SUPPLEMENTARY READING

Braun, K. L., Pietsch, J. H., & Blanchette, P. L. (Eds.). (2000). *Cultural issues in end-of-life decision making.* Thousand Oaks, CA: Sage.

Goelitz, A. (2001). Nurturing life with dreams: Therapeutic dream work with cancer patients. *Clinical Social Work Journal, 29*(4), 375–385.

Hillyer, B. (1993). *Feminism and disability.* Norman: University of Oklahoma Press.

Juarez, G., Ferrell, B., & Borneman, T. (1998). Influence of culture on cancer pain management in Hispanic patients. *Cancer Practice, 6*(5), 262–269.

Kuhl, D. (2002). *What dying people want: Practical wisdom for the end of life.* New York: PublicAffairs.

McLaughlin, L. A., & Braun, K. L. (1998). Asian and Pacific Islander cultural values: Considerations for health care decision making. *Health and Social Work, 23*(2), 116–126.

Sherbourne, C. D., Hays, R. D., Fleishman, J. A., Vitiello, B., Magruder, K. M., Bing, E. G., et al. (2000). Impact of psychiatric conditions on health-related quality of life in persons with HIV infection. *American Journal of Psychiatry, 157,* 248–254.

Siriwardena, A. N., & Clark, D. H. (2004). End-of-life care for ethnic minority groups. *Clinical Cornerstone, 6*(1), 43–48.

Sodergren, S. C., & Hyland, M. E. (2000). What are the positive consequences of illness? *Psychology and Health, 15,* 85–97.

Sormanti, M., & August, J. (1997). Parental bereavement: Spiritual connections with deceased children. *American Journal of Orthopsychiatry, 67*(3), 460–469.

Sourkes, B. M. (1982). *The deepening shade: Psychological aspects of life-threatening illness.* Pittsburgh: University of Pittsburgh Press.

Treisman, G. J., Angelino, A. F., & Hutton, H. E. (2001). Psychiatric issues in the management of patients with HIV infection. *Journal of the American Medical Association, 286*(22), 2857–2864.

Walsh-Burke, K. (2004). Assessing mental health risk in end-of-life care. In J. Berzoff & P. Silverman (Eds.), *Living with dying: A handbook for end-of-life healthcare practitioners* (pp. 360–379). New York: Columbia University Press.

Wendell, S. (1996). *The rejected body: Feminist philosophical reflections on disability.* New York: Routledge.

West, H. F., Engelberg, R. A., Wenrich, M. D., & Curtis, J. R. (2005). Expressions of nonabandonment during the intensive care unit family conference. *Journal of Palliative Medicine, 8*(4), 797–807.

White, D. B., & Curtis, J. R. (2005). Care near the end-of-life in critically ill patients: A North American perspective. *Current Opinions in Critical Care, 11*(6), 610–615.

Wong-Kim, E., & Bloom, J. R. (2005). Depression experienced by young women newly diagnosed with breast cancer. *Psycho-oncology, 14,* 564–573.

Wylie, M. S., & Markowitz, L. M. (1992, September/October). Walking the wire. *The Family Therapy Networker.*

34

Biomedical Ethics

Gary Stein

COURSE DESCRIPTION

Biomedical Ethics is offered as a general introduction to the many ethical issues and dilemmas confronting health-care providers and patients today. The emphasis will be on clinical issues and case studies, including end-of-life care, health-care decision making, the relationship between the health-care professional and patient, and research.

REQUIRED TEXTS

Fins, J. F., &. Maltby, B. S. (2003). *Fidelity, wisdom, and love: Patients and proxies in partnership*. New York: Weill Medical College of Cornell University.

Levine, C. (2006). *Taking sides: Clashing views on controversial bioethical issues* (11th ed.). Guilford, CT: Dushkin.

Mappes, T. A., & DeGrazia, D. (2006). *Biomedical ethics* (6th ed.). Boston: McGraw-Hill.

LEARNING OBJECTIVES

The goal of this course is for students to

- Become familiar with ethical principles used to support moral decision making in today's health-care environment
- Develop critical thinking skills allowing analysis of ethical issues in clinical situations and the formulation of recommendations based upon ethical principles and reasoned moral debate
- Increase awareness and sensitivity to issues involving cultural diversity, personal beliefs, and individual and community values regarding medical treatment decisions
- Think about ethical issues from divergent perspectives and develop their own perspectives based on an analytic process

COURSE OUTLINE

Session 1 Introduction to biomedical ethics
Review of course requirements
What is bioethics?
Ethical decision making

Reading: Mappes & DeGrazia, pp. 26–53

Session 2 Ethical principles in a medical context
Sources of conflict in modern medicine
Bioethics committees: Roles and responsibilities

Discussion:
Levine, Issue 17: Does military necessity override medical ethics?
Levine, Issue 18: Should performance-enhancing drugs be banned from sports?

Reading: Mappes & DeGrazia, pp. 59–72

Session 3 Physician-patient relationship
Informed consent
Truth telling
Medical paternalism

Discussion: Levine, Issue 6: Should truth telling depend on the patient's culture?

Reading: Mappes & DeGrazia, pp. 302–312, 330–334, 340–349

Session 4 Defining death
Forgoing life-sustaining treatments
Futility

Discussion: Levine, Issue 7: Should doctors be able to refuse demands for "futile" treatment?

Reading:
Mappes & DeGrazia, pp. 350–365
Eisenberg, D. (2005, April 4). Lessons of the Schiavo battle. *Time,* pp. 22–33.

Session 5 Deciding for others / surrogate decision making
Capacity to make decisions
Advance directives and respect for autonomy
Artificial nutrition and hydration

Discussion: Levine, Issue 1: Is informed consent still central to medical ethics?

Session 6 Midterm exam

Reading:
Cloud, J. (2000 September 18). A kindler, gentler death. *Time,* pp. 60–74.
Didion, J. (2005). *The year of magical thinking*. New York: Knopf, pp. 3–33.
Fins & Maltby (2003)
Complete advance directives

Session 7 Principles of palliative care
Hospice care
Your own advance directives

Discussion: Levine, Issue 4: Are some advance directives too risky for patients?

Reading: Mappes & DeGrazia, pp. 377–384, 404–413

Session 8 Physician-assisted suicide
Euthanasia

Discussion: Levine, Issue 5: Should physicians be allowed to assist in patient suicide?

Reading: Mappes & DeGrazia, pp. 292–210

Session 9 Family interests in medical decisions
Cochlear implants
Clinical management of intersex infants and children

Discussion: Levine, Issue 2: Can family interests ethically outweigh patient autonomy?

Reading: Mappes & DeGrazia, pp. 224–240, 247–251, 266–271

Session 10 Clinical research
Standards for human research
Use of animals in research

Discussion:
Levine, Issue 12: Should the federal government fund human stem cell research?
Levine, Issue 14: Should animal experimentation be permitted?

Reading: Berg, A. L., Herb, A., & Hurst, M. (2005). Cochlear implants in children. *Journal of Clinical Ethics, 16*(3), 239–250.

Session 11 Guest lecturers

Session 12 Cultural issues in health care

Discussion:

Levine, Issue 10: Should adolescents make their own life-and-death decisions?

Levine, Issue 11: Do parents harm their children when they refuse medical treatment on religious grounds?

Session 13 Research presentations

Session 14 Research presentations

Session 15 Research presentations

35

AIDS and Social Work

Policy and Practice Issues

Susan Taylor-Brown

COURSE DESCRIPTION

Social work has a rich history of responding to society's needy and oppressed. Today, we are facing a pandemic of acquired immunodeficiency syndrome (AIDS), which has major implications for social workers in all practice settings. People with HIV/AIDS experience discrimination in almost every aspect of society, including housing, employment, law enforcement, education, and medical care.

We are beginning to understand the impact that AIDS has not only on the people who have AIDS but on extended family members, significant others, and community. The HIV virus is differentially affecting ethnic/racial/cultural groups in the United States. Each of these groups is responding uniquely to this illness. Therefore, when one is planning and providing services, diversity factors must be taken into account.

This course is designed to provide in-depth knowledge about HIV/AIDS and to produce social workers who will provide community leadership. The course will assist the student in becoming more comfortable working with individuals who are infected with HIV/AIDS. The seminar will use a combination of approaches: lectures, class discussion, films, and presentations by community providers and individuals affected by HIV/AIDS. The seminar will help students become more aware of: (1) the medical realities of HIV/AIDS, (2) the psychosocial implications of the illness as related to treatment issues, (3) the policy issues relevant to the illness, (4) methods of prevention, (5) issues related to professional practice with persons who test positive for HIV, and (6) program planning issues from program design to implementation. The course will teach students to provide culturally sensitive services to individuals infected with HIV/AIDS and other individuals affected by HIV/AIDS.

COURSE OBJECTIVES

Students will be able to:

- Articulate the medical aspects of HIV and related illnesses such as TB
- Identify the psychosocial needs of people with HIV/AIDS, family members, significant others, and the community
- Articulate a plan for implementing programs for people with HIV/AIDS and their significant others from prevention to post-death interventions
- Analyze social policies and legislation related to AIDS, particularly regarding issues of civil rights and discrimination.
- Articulate the differential impact of HIV/AIDS on diverse populations and the relationship of poverty to the differential incidence and prevalence rates as it is experienced worldwide
- Articulate their personal values and attitudes toward HIV/AIDS and examine their relationship to professional practice
- Critically review quantitative and qualitative HIV/AIDS studies with emphasis on the ethical issues involved in doing research with vulnerable populations

Liberal arts perspective: Students are expected to access knowledge acquired throughout their educational experience to guide their involvement in this course. In completing assignments, students will draw on scholarly works across academic disciplines including sociology, philosophy, psychology, history, political science, and economics.

Professional purpose and values: Developing professional social work values and a professional knowledge base is the key goal for this class. The professional skills needed to understand and work with and within the context of individuals, families, and groups are emphasized in this course. These skills include application of theory to assessment and intervention, professional presentation of material, and increased cultural competence.

Social and economic justice: This course pays special attention to how intentional and unintentional forms of social and economic injustice affect and influence human behavior in the social context.

Human diversity and vulnerable populations: Readings, lectures, class discussions, and assignments include content on vulnerable populations. Vulnerable persons are those who are intentionally or unintentionally discriminated against because of one or more attributes or statuses that are not valued by dominant society. Vulnerable persons are at risk of social isolation and economic disadvantage and its consequences because of the pervasive effects of structural inequality and lack of power.

REQUIRED TEXTS

Behrman, G. (2004). *The invisible people: How the U. S. has slept through the global AIDS pandemic, the greatest humanitarian catastrophe of our time.* New York: Free Press.

SUPPLEMENTAL TEXTS

Aronstein, D. M., & Thompson, B. J. (Eds.). (1998). *HIV and social work: A practitioner's guide.* New York: Harrington Park Press.

Farmer, P., Connors, M., & Simmons, J. (2005). *Women, poverty, and AIDS: Sex, drugs, and structural violence.* Boston: Common Courage Press.

Lynch, V. (Ed.). (1999). *HIV/AIDS at year 2000: A sourcebook for social workers.* Boston: Allyn and Bacon

Mann, J., & Tarantola, D. (1996). *AIDS in the world II.* New York: Oxford University Press.

Wyatt-Morley, C. (1997). *AIDS memoir: Journal of an HIV-positive mother.* West Hartford, CT: Kumarian Press.

REQUIREMENTS

Class participation: Students are expected to have read the assigned readings and to participate in class discussion. Students are encouraged to consider the applicability of the readings to their practice. There will be opportunities for individual and group presentations of assignments.

Assignments: Students are expected to complete three assignments: a commentary, a personal accounts paper, and service learning.

Commentary: Students are to write three 250-word reaction papers on the class readings and seminar presentations in which they explore a topic that they find provocative and provide an analysis. Discussions questions will be provided for each session, and students may select the ones to which they wish to respond. Students are to critically examine a specific aspect of the readings, not just describe what they have read.

Personal accounts: Students may read either Wyatt-Morley's memoir or a personal account of your choice. (Other texts may be selected with instructor permission.) Students will write a reaction paper on the book they choose, in which they identify the key issues the person dealt with and their own reactions to those issues. Students should reflect on how this knowledge and their reaction to it will affect their social work practice. This paper should be two to three pages long.

Service learning options: Students will participate in a service learning option. For example, they may choose to help orphaned youths prepare for the GED; explore food donation options; investigate community opportunities for fund-raising, design a program, and implement it; or develop a guide of available summer programs, collect camp applications, and organize a resource file. In order to do this, students must meet with the instructor during the first three weeks of the semester to develop an individualized plan. Students are welcome to work with another student. Service learning projects will incorporate a logic model, and students will write a reflective piece regarding the experience. Students will present a summary of their project in seminar and write the following reflection pieces:

1. Beginning-of-semester reflection essay: Review the course objectives and respond to the following questions: Which objectives are you most comfortable with? Which objectives are you the least comfortable with? Explain why you think this is the case.
2. Middle-of-semester reflection essay: Write about the growth you have observed regarding the course objectives. Which are you the most comfortable with now?
3. End-of-semester reflection essay: What strategies did you use to overcome your fears and assumptions? What biases did you bring to the seminar? How does this learning affect your social work practice skills? As you review the course objectives, which are you the most comfortable with? Which are you the least comfortable with? Why? Finally, how could this experience be improved?

COURSE OUTLINE

Session 1 Overview of HIV/AIDS: The intersection of medical and social realities

Learning about HIV/AIDS stigma and misinformation: Select two people to talk with about HIV. Try to pick one person from your work network and one from your personal network. Explore the following questions with them: What do you know about HIV/AIDS? Who gets HIV/AIDS in the United States? Is it as big a problem now as it was in the 1990s? How would you feel about working with a person who is HIV positive? What worries you about HIV? Take notes regarding their areas of concern, their misconceptions, and their attitudes toward people who are HIV positive. Try to educate each individual if he or she has misperceptions. Then the class will compare experiences.

Media analysis: For a week, keep track of mentions of HIV/AIDS in articles, news reports, and television shows. Also take note of AIDS benefits that appear in print or are discussed on the radio or on television, and search the Web for recent HIV/AIDS information. Note the dates of the publications and the subjects covered. For example, do articles discussing AIDS orphans talk about AIDS orphans in the United States or just Africa and Asia?

Sessions 2 and 3

AIDS: Diagnosis and treatment
Film: *A Closer Walk*
Epidemiology of HIV with emphasis on the disproportionate impact on different ethnic/cultural groups
Scientific paradigms: How much do we know?
At-risk behaviors versus at-risk populations
Disease characteristics
Transmission: Sexually transmitted diseases
Screening tests: False positives and negatives
Treatment modalities: Protease inhibitors, vaccine trials, clinical treatment trials
Course of illness
TB: The intersection of two epidemics
Global overview: A powerful HIV/AIDS pandemic

Required reading:
Aronstein & Thompson, section 1 (pp. 3–74)
Behrman, preface, chapters 1–6
Farmer, Connors, & Simmons, introduction, parts 1–3
Lynch, chapter 1
Mann & Tarantola, chapters 1, 10–12
Wyatt-Morley or personal account approved by instructor
Visit the Center for Disease Control's Web site (www.cdc.gov). Find information regarding HIV/AIDS incidence and prevalence in the United States and in your state and city.

Sessions 4 and 5

Social construction of AIDS in society
Commentary due session 4
Personal account paper due session 5

Reflecting on a career: Personal narrative presented by a social worker who has provided HIV/AIDS services in the community
Stigma/discrimination
The impact of marginalization on people with HIV/AIDS
The differential impact on communities of color, injecting drug users and their partners, and gay men
Fear: AFRAIDS
Parental loss due to AIDS
Stigmatization of family and caregivers

Following a lecture in which current information regarding the psychosocial research literature is provided, the class will meet with a person who is HIV positive or a family member of someone who is. He or she will share his or her experiences with the group, and we will examine the service implications. Additionally, service providers who are working with infected parents will discuss the challenges of permanency planning.

Session 6 Care for the professional caregiver
Midsemester assessment due

Stigmatization of the professional who is associated with a stigmatized group
Need for support
Risk in the health-care workplace
Worker's responsibility to serve AIDS patient
Health-care team formation
Fear
Family pressures
Morale
Image
Interdisciplinary care: Team dynamics, working with colleagues who are HIV positive
Care for professional caregivers

These sessions will help students to provide service to HIV-infected and -affected individuals. There are unique dynamics related to the pandemic that affect our ability to provide care.

Required reading:
Aronstein & Thompson, section 5 (pp. 527–560); section 2, part B (pp. 165–302); section 3, part A (pp. 315–386)
Zibalese-Crawford, M., Brennan, J. P., & Stein, J. *Assessing the social work response to HIV/AIDS.* Washington, DC: National Association of Social Workers Task Force on HIV/AIDS.

Sessions 7–11 The continuum of care for those infected with HIV
Policy and practice implications
Service learning projects due session 9

Practice:
Case management
Prevention
Acute care
Long-term care
Care for caregivers

Policy issues:
Orphans: Transitional services
Needle exchange

Condom distribution in high schools and in jails
Mandatory testing and Fourth Amendment issues
Testing of health-care workers

Legal issues:
Risks and responsibilities
Labor law and liability
Presidential and congressional AIDS commissions
Funding issues
Agency policies
Ethical issues

The last two sessions will combine key policy issues with treatment issues. Various community providers will share their experiences with the class. Students will present their service learning projects to the class.

Required reading
Pequegnat & Szapocznik
Working Committee on HIV, Children and Families (chapters and due dates TBA)

Recommended reading:
Aronstein & Thompson, pp. 483–510
Farmer, Connors, & Simmons, chapters 8 and 9
Lynch, chapters 5, 8, 10, 12, 13, 15–18
Mann & Tarantola, chapter 29

Session 12 Course wrap-up

USEFUL WEB SITES

AIDS Alliance: http://www.aids-alliance.org/
Centers for Disease Control: http://www.cdc.gov/
Children Affected By AIDS Foundation: http://www.caaf4kids.org
Child Welfare League of America: http://www.cwla.org/
Health Resources Administration: http://www.ask.hrsa.gov/HIV.cfm
Kaiser Family Foundation: http://www.kff.org/youthhivstds/index.cfm

Part Nine

Specialty Programs

36

University of Iowa, School of Social Work

Susan Murty

The School of Social Work has developed an innovative program to train social workers for practice in end-of-life services with initial funding from the Project on Death in America. The coursework prepares students for practice in hospice programs and in hospital social work in pediatric and adult oncology, palliative care units, and other social work settings focused on the needs of individuals at the end of life, their families, and other bereaved individuals. It is based on the family-centered and community-based principles that permeate the entire curriculum in the MSW program. End-of-life services are based on the values of the hospice movement, which include an emphasis on patient-directed treatment, services focused on the family as well as the patient, pain control and palliative care, a continuum of services available in the home and in inpatient settings, and integrated services provided by an interdisciplinary team and focused on medical, social, and spiritual needs.

APPROVED ELECTIVES IN THE SCHOOL OF SOCIAL WORK

*42:254	Introductory Seminar in End-of-Life Care in Rural Communities	3 s.h.
*42:271	Independent Study associated with completing hospice volunteer training (may be completed without academic credit)	1 s.h.
*42:255	Integrative Seminar in End-of-Life Care	1 s.h.

Students select six hours from the following list of approved electives:

42:253	Survey of Gerontological Programs and Services	3 s.h.
42:194	SW Practice in Health Care Settings	2 s.h.
42:219	Aging and the Family	2–3 s.h.
42:281	Interventions in End-of-Life Care	2–3 s.h.

42:224	Spirituality and Ethics in Social Work Practice	2–3 s.h.
42:281	Social Work Theory and Practice in Long-Term Care	2 s.h.
42:281	Death, Dying, and Bereavement (cross-listed with Aging Studies)	2 s.h.
42:281	Grief Therapy	2 s.h.
42:281	Social Work in Rural Communities	3 s.h.

Note: Students choose courses from the list of electives in consultation with their academic advisor and the coordinator of the end-of-life care field of practice. The courses marked with an asterisk are required core courses in the end-of-life field of practice. These courses may be open to other students with permission of the instructor, but students in end-of-life care have priority. MSW students normally take twelve semester hours of electives. Students who have already completed hospice volunteer training or have considerable hospice experience may discuss waiving the hospice volunteer training with permission of the coordinator of the end-of-life care field of practice.

ELECTIVES OFFERED IN OTHER DEPARTMENTS

32:163 Introduction to Biomedical Ethics (Department of Religious Studies, cross-listed in Aging Studies)

32:193 Death, Dying, and Tradition (Department of Religion Studies, cross-listed in Aging Studies)

SEQUENCE OF COURSEWORK FOR FIELD OF PRACTICE IN END-OF-LIFE CARE

Semester	Courses
Year 1: Fall semester	Introductory Seminar in End-of-Life Care in Rural Communities
Year 1: Spring semester	Foundation practicum
	Hospice volunteer training as independent study (if needed)
Summer semester	Electives related to end-of-life care
Year 2: Fall semester	Advanced practicum in end-of-life care
Year 2: Spring semester	Advanced practicum in end-of-life care
	Integrative seminar in end-of-life care

SOME ADVANCED PRACTICUM SITES

Iowa City Hospice (serves seven county rural region with office in Iowa City; placements both in hospice social work and bereavement programs)

Washington Hospice

Cedar Valley Hospice

Holden Comprehensive Cancer Center, University Of Iowa Health Care: Adult Oncology, Pediatric Oncology, Palliative Care, Social Services (serves the state of Iowa, and some patients from surrounding states)

Veterans Administration Medical Center, Iowa City and Des Moines (serve veterans from large rural region)

West Liberty Retirement Community (provides skilled nursing, assisted living, and independent living services in West Liberty)

Hospice Program at Oakdale Correctional Facility and other facilities

Hospice of Central Iowa and other hospices in the Des Moines area and surrounding rural region

37

Life Transitions

Working with End-of-Life Relationships

Denice Goodrich Liley

WORKSHOP DESCRIPTION

Death is an emotional challenge for most individuals and families. This workshop takes an interdisciplinary approach to death, the process of dying, and end-of-life care to examine the ethical, sociological, medical, psychological, legal, political, metaphysical, and religious issues that come up for individuals and their families. Attention will be given to the impact of end of life on relationships and strategies of intervention.

WORKSHOP GOALS

The goal of this workshop is for students:

- To gain an appreciation of death, end of life, and the process of dying as natural components of the life span, and to appreciate how an awareness of mortality contributes to the construction of meaning in one's life
- To understand death, end of life, and the process of dying from a multidimensional, multidisciplinary perspective, and to appreciate how culture, history, and individual differences contribute to the understanding of, preparation for, and coping with end of life
- To become acquainted with theoretical, scientific, and practical knowledge relevant to end of life, death, grief, and bereavement, and to integrate that knowledge in order to facilitate personal growth and development

SKILL DEVELOPMENT GOALS

By the end of the workshop, participants will be able to:

- Identify their own feelings and attitudes about death and dying
- Identify various perspectives of palliative care and end-of-life care, including those of health-care providers, family, children, and patients
- Identify resources necessary for coping with end-of-life and palliative care for patients, family members, and significant others
- Discuss the psychosocial and communication issues involved in palliative care and end-of-life care for care providers, families, and patients
- Apply specific skills to assist the patient, family, and care providers in creating a therapeutic climate for palliative and end-of-life care

REQUIRED TEXTS

Callanan, M., & Kelley, P. (1997). *Final gifts.* New York: Bantam Books.

The text should be read prior to the beginning of the workshop.

RECOMMENDED TEXTS

DeSpelder, L. A., & Strickland, A. L. (2005). *The last dance: Encountering death and dying* (7th ed.). New York: McGraw-Hill.
Kübler-Ross, E. (1970). *On death and dying.* New York: Macmillian.

WORKSHOP SCHEDULE

Session 1 Overview of workshop format and expectations
Introductions
Group exercise: "Death brings to mind"
Process group experience
Didactic information
Just what is death?
Exposure and encounters with death
Harvard criteria for death
Context of dying care
Group activity: Workshop participants will be divided into groups of eight participants. Each group will be given a large sheet of colored butcher paper (three-by-five feet) and a box of crayons. The group is to write words and/or phrases and draw symbols they think of that represent death. The group

is given forty-five minutes to do this activity. Each group should discuss their personal experiences with end of life among themselves as they do the activity. Groups will then present their experiences to the whole workshop. The papers will be hung up around the room and remain there throughout the workshop.

Homework: Each participant will be given an index card at the end of the session. Participants will be asked to write two or three questions for the funeral director for the next session. The index cards will be collected when participants arrive at the funeral home the next day.

Reading:

Candib, L. M. (2002). Truth telling and advance planning at the end of life: Problems with autonomy in a multicultural world. *Families, Systems, and Health, 20*(3), 213–227.

Duhanamel, F., & Dupuis, F. (2003). Families in palliative care: Exploring family and health-care professionals' beliefs. *International Journal of Palliative Nursing, 9*(3), 113–119.

Kagawa-Singer, M., & Blackhall, L. J. (2001). Negotiating cross-cultural issues at the end of life: "You got to go where he lives." *Journal of the American Medical Association, 286*(23), 2993–3001.

Werth, J. L. (2002). Legal and ethical considerations for mental health professionals related to end-of-life care and decision making. *American Behaviorist, 46*(3), 373–388.

Session 2 Meet at funeral home
Review of index cards
Answer questions
Introduction and discussion
Co-facilitation by funeral director
How funeral directors are involved with families
Funeral services
Legal issues
Body dispositions (cremation, burial, memorialization)
Tour of facility
Caskets, grave markers, grave liners, urns
Crematorium
Question-and-answer session

Guest panel: Three to five religious representatives from the community will discuss common experiences and themes they have witnessed with individuals and families in the process of dying and end-of-life care as it relates to spirituality, faith, and religion. This discussion will give participants the opportunity to explore the challenges of meeting diverse individual and family needs in end-of-life care.

Question-and-answer session

Session 3

Process previous session
Dying trajectories
Breaking bad news
Truth telling and disclosure
Grief and bereavement
Cultural influences

Group activity: Small groups of three to five participants will each be given a different case study related to end of life, death, or the process of dying. The case studies should address issues related to culture, age, gender, and life span, such as a young Hispanic couple whose child dies of SIDS, a single mother who is a devoted Catholic whose adult child dies in a car accident caused by a drunk driver, an individual with ALS who is in a committed same-sex relationship, a forty-five-year-old woman with terminal breast cancer, an elderly woman in need of hospice services, and an Alaskan Native man in a nursing home whose prognosis is terminal. Case studies will give a small amount of information about the person and the end-of-life issues with which he or she is dealing. Groups are to address their perceptions of key issues for the case study and what things need to be considered. Each group is to formulate an action plan of things that need to be done. Groups will spend about forty-five minutes on the case studies and will then report back to the entire workshop. The workshop will then discuss not only the case studies but also the groups' interactions while they worked.

Homework: None

Session 4

Film: *Dying in America* (Moyers)
Discussion of selected film segments
Relate film content and workshop experiences
Discussion

- Mindful living
- Five Wishes
- Self-determination
- Advance directives
- Living will
- Durable power of health care
- Community resources

Hospice (adult and child)
Bereavement services
Obituaries
Healing activities

Group activity: Participants return to same small groups used for for previous session. Each group is given a large sheet of paper with which to make a collage that they feel represents their life and what is important to them. Magazines, markers, glue, and other craft supplies will be available. Groups will spend about forty-five minutes on the collage and will discuss the collages among themselves. The entire workshop group will then discuss the process, with a focus on relating our living to our process of dying

Answer last-minute questions
Review assignments for students seeking credit
Evaluation: Endings

REQUIREMENTS

Participants must attend all lectures, discussions, and activity sessions. Active participation in all classroom discussions and simulations is required. Each participant must write a narrative reaction to the weekend workshop reflecting on his or her individual experiences at the workshop and answering the following questions: What was your experience in this workshop? Was it what you expected? Did the workshop bring up things you had not thought of before? Participants must conduct an interview with a family member or significant other concerning his or her wishes for his or her end-of-life care, funeral, and burial and write a paper detailing the interview, the participant's relationship to the person interviewed, what he or she learned from the interview, what was helpful, and any other relevant insights obtained. The interview should be no longer than four word-processed pages. Graduate students are required to complete an annotated bibliography of five articles related to end of life and their individual study major.

BIBLIOGRAPHY

Albom, M. (1997). *Tuesdays with Morrie: An old man, a young man, and life's greatest lesson*. New York: Doubleday.

Baker, M. J. (2000). Knowledge and attitudes of health care social workers regarding advance directives. *Social Work in Health Care, 32,* 61–74.

Bertman, S. L. (1999). *Grief and the healing arts.* Amityville, NY: Baywood.

Braun, K. L., Pietsch, J. H., & Blanchette, P. L. (2000). *Cultural issues in end-of-life decision making.* Thousand Oaks, CA: Sage.

Buckman, R. (1988). *I don't know what to say.* Toronto: Key Porter Books.

Candib, L. M. (2002). Truth telling and advance planning at the end of life: Problems with autonomy in a multicultural world. *Families, Systems, and Health, 20,* 213–228.

Coberly, M. (2002). *Sacred passage: How to provide fearless, compassionate care.* Boston: Shambhala Publications.

Davidson, J., & Doka, K. J. (1999). *Living with grief: At work, at school, at worship.* Washington, DC: Brunner/Mazel.

Davies, B., et. al. (1995). *Fading away: The experience of transition in families with terminal illness.* Amityville, NY: Baywood.

Davies, R. (2003). Establishing need for palliative care services for children/young people. *British Journal of Nursing, 12,* 224–232.

Duhamel, F., & Dupuis, F. (2003). Families in palliative care: Exploring family and health-care professionals' beliefs. *International Journal of Palliative Nursing, 9,* 113–119.

Ekblad, S., Marttila, A., & Emilsson, M. (2000). Cultural challenges in end-of-life care: Reflections from focus groups' interviews with hospice staff in Stockholm. *Journal of Advanced Nursing, 31,* 623–631.

Enes, S. P. (2003). An exploration of dignity in palliative care. *Palliative Medicine, 17,* 263–269.

Estess, J. (2004). *Tales from the bed: On living, dying, and having it all.* New York: Atria Books.

Fulghum, R. (1995). *From beginning to end: Rituals of our lives.* New York: Villard Books.

Hallenbeck, J. (1999). Decisions at the end-of-life: Cultural considerations beyond medical ethics. *Generations, 23,* 24–30.

Harris, J. W. (2000). *Remembrances and celebrations: A book of eulogies, letters, and epitaphs.* New York: Random House.

Jenkins, M. L. (2002). *You only die once: Planning for the end of life with grace and gusto.* Brentwood, TN: Integrity Publishing.

Jones, C. (1997). *R.I.P.: The complete book of death and dying.* New York: HarperCollins.

Kessler, D. (1997). *The rights of the dying: A companion for life's final moments.* New York: HarperCollins.

Klug, M. B., Gessert, C., & Forbes, S. (2001). The need to revise assumptions about the end of life: Implications for social work practice. *Health and Social Work, 26,* 38–48.

Kübler-Ross, E. (1969). *On death and dying.* New York: Collier Books.

Kübler-Ross, E., & Kessler, D. (2000). *Life lessons: Two experts on death and dying teach us about the mysteries of life and living.* New York: Scribner.

Kushner, H. S. (1981). *When bad things happen to good people.* New York: Avon.

Lewis, C. S. (1961). *A grief observed.* New York: Bantam Books.

Lynch, T. (1997). *The undertaking: Life studies from the dismal trade.* New York: W. W. Norton.

Morris, V. (2002). *Talking about death won't kill you.* New York: Workman Press.

Nuland, S. B. (1994). *How we die: Reflections on life's final chapter.* New York: Knopf.

O'Gorman, S. M. (1998). Death and dying in contemporary society: An evaluation of current attitudes and the rituals associated with death and dying and their relevance to recent understandings of health and healing. *Journal of Advanced Nursing, 6,* 1127–1135.

Remen, R. N. (1996). *Kitchen table wisdom: Stories that heal.* New York: Riverhead Books/Putnam.

Rinpoche, S. (1992). *The Tibetan book of living and dying.* San Francisco: Harper.

Singer, M. K., & Blackhall, L. J. (2001). Negotiating cross-cultural issues at the end of life: "You got to go where he lives." *Journal of the American Medical Association, 286*(23), 2993–3001.

Sontag, S. (1978). *Illness as a metaphor.* New York: Farrar, Straus and Giroux.

Stone, R. (1997). *The healing art of storytelling: A sacred journey of personal discovery.* New York: Hyperion.

Weber, J. A., & Fournier, D. G. (1985). Family support and a child's adjustment to death. *Family Relations, 34,* 43–49.

Werth, J. L. (2002). Legal and ethical considerations for mental health care professions related to end-of-life care and decision making. *American Behaviorial Scientist, 46,* 373–388.

38

Smith College/Baystate Medical Center End-of-Life Care Certificate Program

Joan Berzoff

There are growing numbers of individuals and families in need of end-of-life care—children, adolescents, and adults who are chronically ill or have life-limiting conditions such as cancer, heart disease, renal disease, and AIDS. Many are being kept alive through new technologies. As the population ages, there are more elderly individuals with progressive chronic disabilities. In addition, there are people in community shelters and psychiatric institutions and others who are homeless or in prisons who are also facing death. Never before have clinical social work interventions been more needed. The terminally ill person, his or her family and social supports, health-care providers, and the clergy all benefit from the skills of the clinical social work practitioner.

To date, clinical social workers have been ill prepared at the masters level to effectively address the needs of those facing the end of life. In 2000, the Open Society Institute's Project on Death in America provided Dr. Joan Berzoff a Social Work Leadership Award to develop an advanced practice certificate program in end-of-life care for clinical social workers. To date, ninety post-masters social workers have been trained to lead in shaping the culture of dying in America by writing grants, making systems changes in their institutions, publishing articles, teaching or supervising in schools for social work, and developing new programs.

PROGRAM STRUCTURE

Designed for clinicians with between two and five years of postgraduate clinical experience who are currently working with end-of-life care issues, this program consists of two weekend periods of intensive coursework, punctuated by a six-month clinical internship in which students work on a weekly basis with three clinical study cases (patients and families) and lead one group in their work setting. Students also develop or join a monthly interdisciplinary peer supervision team and apply what they learn to their practices. The end-of-life certificate program carries 50.5 continuing education credits. Students will receive two hours of telephonic clinical supervision each month either from advanced social work supervisors at Cancer Care, Inc., a nationally recognized expert in end-of-life clinical practice, or from other outstanding supervisors closely associated with the program. At the end of the internship, students write a final paper related to clinical theory, practice, and/or leadership.

PROGRAM FOCUS AREAS

The following curriculum is offered twice a year:

Psychodynamic Views on End-of-Life Care
This seminar covers theories that address loss, separation, attachment, death, and bereavement. Freud's concept of identification; Bowlby's, Spitz's, and Mahler's contributions to understanding loss and growth; and current attachment theorists are presented.

Clinical Practice
This case-based seminar addresses issues of death and dying and bereavement over the life cycle. The trajectory of illness; developmental issues for children, adolescents, and adults; transference and countertransference; and uses of self are addressed.

Diversity and Disadvantage in End-of-Life Care
Cultural and economic factors play a significant part in health care, health-care decision making, and end-of-life experiences. This class will review cultural competency standards in end-of-life practice and consider the influence of culture, ethnicity, and economic disadvantage on attitudes and beliefs about death and dying.

Ethical Issues in End-of-Life Care
This seminar addresses ethical issues in interdisciplinary palliative care, hospice, and bereavement. Patient autonomy, advance directives, physician-assisted suicide, and cessation of life supports are discussed in case examples.

Grieving Children and Their Families: Relational Issues in a Developmental Context
This seminar addresses how death, grief, and bereavement shape self and identity. Using research drawn from work with children and adolescents, this course challenges concepts of "normal" grief, and alternative views of grief and bereavement are presented.

Spiritual Dimensions of End-of-Life Care
The intersection of spiritual and psychodynamic issues at the end of life is addressed. How multicultural and ethnic groups view death, dying, and grieving is included, and their implications for practice are discussed.

Professional Caregiving in End-of-Life Care
This seminar offers a theoretical framework within which to examine the experiences of professional caregivers alongside the experiences of patients and families. Videotaped interviews with a bereaved family and health-care professionals will be used to elaborate on ethnographic perspectives on professional caregiving and clinical practice in end-of-life care.

Clinical Practice II
This seminar uses participants' cases to discuss uses of self, countertransference, and intersubjective practice in palliative, hospice, and bereavement practices. Participants consider the intersection of psychological, developmental, existential, and spiritual issues in advanced clinical practice. Interdisciplinary support, education, and supervision are considered. One hour of this seminar provides an opportunity for participants to present their case studies and to teach and educate other members of the class in a seminar designed to look at advanced uses of self.

Leadership in End-of-Life Care
This seminar covers the use of self as teacher, ethical decision maker, program developer, advocate, consultant, and policy maker in end-of-life care.

Advanced Spirituality Seminar
This seminar will expand students' knowledge and skills in integrating psychological and spiritual ways of making meaning. Special attention will be given to applying knowledge from a variety of religious traditions and spiritual disciplines to a range of end-of-life settings. The seminar is designed to enrich the practitioner's own comfort with diverse religious and spiritual practices.

Current Issues in Hospice and Palliative Care
This seminar introduces core issues in palliative care and the history of the hospice movement. Clinical and systems issues and current challenges facing the movement as well as the issues of race and ethnic, spiritual, existential, and psychological practices are discussed.

Lesbians and Gay Men at the End of Their Lives
Participants will learn about barriers to disclosure of sexual orientation in health care, interventions to assist lesbians and gay men with health-care decision making and end-of-life care planning, and the role of social workers

in dealing with issues of transference and countertransference in working with this population.

Complex Legal and Public Policy Issues
Advance directives, physician-assisted suicide, the cessation of life support, and other legal and ethical issues are discussed, drawing on considerations from the first session and clinical internships.

Pain and Symptom Management
This seminar will review the psychosocial components of comprehensive pain assessment and management. Special attention will be given to interventions for patients and families, barriers, and misconceptions, as well as cultural, ethical, and medical issues. Advocacy and policy implications and the role of the social worker in pain and symptom management will be considered.

39

New York University Post-Master's Certificate Program

Palliative and End-of-Life Care

Susan Gerbino

WHO SHOULD ATTEND?

Experienced social workers with an MSW degree and a minimum of one year of experience in palliative and end-of-life care work

PROGRAM

This certificate program provides an integrated sequence of courses designed to promote the interaction of theory and practice to enhance the clinician's advanced practice skills. Using a biopsychosocial-spiritual framework, it will allow students to build clinical practice knowledge, expand assessment and clinical intervention skills, examine the assessment and treatment needs of patients and their families, and explore dilemmas in caring rather than curing. It will also provide opportunities for students to develop leadership skills.

CERTIFICATE REQUIREMENTS

In order to earn the certificate, students are required to complete all four courses. Students can complete the courses in one year by taking two courses per semester, or in two years by taking one course per semester. Students may also take courses individually.

Ten CEUs will be awarded for each course completed, and forty for the full program.

COURSES

Multidimensional Perspectives

This course consists of five sessions on ethical issues and five sessions on pain and symptom management. The ethics sessions will offer an in-depth exploration of bioethical principles and their application to patients and families facing life-threatening illnesses. Case examples will be drawn from the students' cases and from classic landmark cases such as Quinlan. The pain management sessions will introduce students to the comprehensive assessment of pain and other symptoms along the continuum of illness and at the end of life. Students will learn to intervene to ease the suffering of both patients and families.

Theories of Attachment, Loss, and Bereavement

This course examines palliative and end-of-life care through attachment, grief, and bereavement theories. A focus on individual relationships with the dying or deceased person will provide a framework for understanding how relationships are changed but not necessarily severed.

Case Seminar

This course is an integrative seminar in which students' cases are used to discuss clinical practice in end-of-life care, including bereavement. The course considers the intersection of theory and practice, including use of self, transference, countertransference, boundary issues, self-disclosure, and ethical-clinical tensions.

Interdisciplinary Collaboration and Leadership Development

This course enables participants to gain leadership mastery and skills in interdisciplinary collaboration. Theories, practice examples, and case presentations will be used to integrate practice and theory.

Part Ten

Other Resources

40

Resource Enrichment Center

Karen Bullock

The Resource Enrichment Center for Improving Care at the End of Life (www.eolresource.htfd.uconn.edu) addresses the need for:

- Continuing education for advanced knowledge and skills in the area of end-of-life care
- Ongoing program innovation and evaluation
- A solid infrastructure of leaders in the field who provide training at the graduate and postgraduate levels

The Resource Enrichment Center offers essential psychosocial supports for terminally ill patients and their families, continuing education for practitioners, and Web-enhanced courses. This resource serves as an arena for collaboration between schools of social work and practice sites that might not otherwise have access to up-to-date research on care for the dying and bereaved. Evaluation results have been used to target, attract, retain, and cultivate graduate students while transforming the educational outcomes for social work leadership in care at the end of life.

41

National Association of Social Workers

Karyn Walsh

The National Association of Social Workers has several educational resources that address palliative and end-of-life care and the social worker's role.

The *NASW Standards for Social Work Practice in Palliative and End of Life Care* offers social workers guidelines for their work in this arena. Social work experts contributed to this important educational tool for social workers who work with individuals receiving palliative or end-of-life care and their loved ones across many practice settings. The standards can be accessed at no charge from http://www.socialworkers.org/practice/bereavement/standards/default.asp.

Understanding End of Life Care: The Social Worker's Role is a Web-based course for social workers practicing with individuals who are affected by life-limiting illness or injury and bereavement. The course covers end-of-life experiences across the continuum of palliative care, dying, death, and bereavement; provides information about dying and death across the life span; and highlights the importance of understanding cultural differences and values surrounding end-of-life care. Social work assessment and intervention strategies are included. The course can be accessed free of charge at http://www.naswwebed.org and offers social workers two free CEUs.

Understanding Cancer: The Social Worker's Role is a Web-based course for social workers on cancer, the care involved, and the social work role with individuals affected by cancer. The course provides information on palliative and end-of-life care, cultural awareness and diversity, and social work intervention skills helpful for practicing with individuals affected by cancer. The course can be accessed free of charge at http://www.naswwebed.org and offers social workers two CEUs.

Contributors

Dorothy S. Becvar
Saint Louis University
School of Social Service

Mercedes Bern-Klug
University of Iowa
School of Social Work

Joan Berzoff
Smith College School for Social Work

Hillel Bodek
Society for Clinical Social Work, Inc.

Cheryl Brandsen
Calvin College
Department of Social Work

Karen Bullock
University of Connecticut
School of Social Work

Mary Carlsen
St. Olaf College
Department of Social Work

Ellen L. Csikai
University of Alabama
School of Social Work

Mark de St. Aubin
University of Utah
College of Social Work

Cynthia Forrest
University of South Carolina
College of Social Work

Cynthia Garthwait
Univeristy of Montana
Department of Social Work

Diane Green
Florida Atlantic University
School of Social Work

Susan Gerbino
New York University
School of Social Work

Helen Harris
Baylor University
School of Social Work

Susan Hedlund
Cancer Care Resources
Oregon Health Sciences University

Barbara Jones
University of Texas–Austin
School of Social Work

Betty J. Kramer
University of Wisconsin–Madison
School of Social Work

Denice Goodrich Liley
Boise State University
School of Social Work

John Linder
University of California–Davis
Cancer Center

Taryn Lindhorst
University of Washington
School of Social Work

Bonnie Letinich
University of Washington
School of Social Work

Jerry Jo Manfred-Gilham
Franciscan University of Steubenville
Department of Social Work

Pamela J. Miller
Portland State University
School of Social Work

Vicki Murdock
University of Wyoming
School of Social Work

Susan Murty
University of Iowa
School of Social Work

Jane Roberts
University of South Florida
School of Social Work

Lucinda Lee Roff
University of Alabama
School of Social Work

Sheila Gillespie Roth
Carlow University
Social Work Department

Sara Sanders
University of Iowa
School of Social Work

Tracy Schroepfer
University of Wisconsin–Madison
School of Social Work

Mary Sormanti
Columbia University
School of Social Work

Gary Stein
Yeshiva University
Wurzweiler School of Social Work

Susan Taylor-Brown
University of Rochester Medical School
Department of Pediatrics

Froma Walsh
University of Chicago

Karyn Walsh
National Association of Social Workers

Katherine Walsh
Springfield College
School of Social Work

Sherri Weisenfluh
Hospice of the Bluegrass